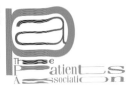

a simple guide to
type 2 diabetes

BESTMEDICINE Health Handbooks

A Simple Guide to Type 2 Diabetes
First published – September 2005

Published by
CSF Medical Communications Ltd
1 Bankside, Lodge Road, Long Hanborough
Oxfordshire, OX29 8LJ, UK
T +44 (0)1993 885370 F +44 (0)1993 881868
enquiries@bestmedicine.com
www.bestmedicine.com
www.csfmedical.com

Editor Dr Eleanor Bull
Medical Editor Dr Eugene Hughes
Creative Director & Project Manager Julia Potterton
Designer Lee Smith
Layout Julie Smith
Publisher Stephen I'Anson

© CSF Medical Communications Ltd 2005

ISBN: 1-905466-02-1

BESTMEDICINE is a trademark of CSF Medical Communications Ltd

contents

ACKNOWLEDGEMENTS

The *BESTMEDICINE Simple Guides* team is very grateful to a number of people who have made this project possible. In particular we'd like to thank Anne Taylor, Jane Cassidy, Caroline Delasalle and Amelie (5 months). Thank you to Ben for his endless enthusiasm, energy and creativity, to Molly (7) and George (5) and of course to Hetta. Julie and Rob who went far beyond the call of duty and Julie's ability to put pages together for hours on end was hugely inspiring.

A Simple Guide to your Health Service

Emma Catherall   Co-ordinator

Advisory Panel

Richard Stevens   GP
Sue Allan   Practice nurse
Kate Emden   Practice nurse
John Reckless   Endocrinologist
Michael Gum   Pharmacist
John Chater   Binley's health and care
                    information specialist
                    www.binleys.com

simple

simple *adj.* **1.** easy to understand or do: *a simple problem.* **2.** plain; unadorned: *a simple dress.* **3.** Not combined or complex: *a simple mechanism.* **4.** Unaffected or unpretentious: *although he became famous he remained a simple man.* **5.** sincere; frank: *a simple explanation was readily accepted.* **6.** (*prenominal*) without additions or modifications: *the witness told the simple truth.*

ABOUT THE AUTHOR

REBECCA FOX-SPENCER

Rebecca Fox-Spencer graduated from Cambridge University with a BA Honours degree in Natural Sciences and then completed a PhD in Neurochemistry at University College London. As well as publishing her own research work internationally, Rebecca has written for other publications in the BESTMEDICINE series. She now lives in South Oxfordshire.

ABOUT THE EDITOR

EUGENE HUGHES

Eugene Hughes is a GP who lives and practises on the Isle of Wight. He was a founder member of Primary Care Diabetes UK and is Chairman of Primary Care Diabetes Europe.

FOREWORD

TRISHA MACNAIR
Doctor and BBC Health Journalist

Getting involved in managing your own medical condition – or helping those you love or care for to manage theirs – is a vital step towards keeping as healthy as possible. Whilst doctors, nurses and the rest of your healthcare team can help you with expert advice and guidance, nobody knows your body, your symptoms and what is right for *you* as well as you do.

There is no long-term (chronic) medical condition or illness that I can think of where the person concerned has absolutely no influence at all on their situation. The way you choose to live your life, from the food you eat to the exercise you take, will impact upon your disease, your well-being and how able you are to cope. You are in charge!

Being involved in making choices about your treatment helps you to feel in control of your problems, and makes sure you get the help that you really need. Research clearly shows that when people living with a chronic illness take an active role in looking after themselves, they can bring about significant improvements in their illness and vastly improve the quality of life they enjoy. Of course, there may be occasions when you feel particularly unwell and it all seems out of your control. Yet most of the time there are plenty of things that you can do in order to reduce the negative effects that your condition can have on your life. This way you feel as good as possible and may even be able to alter the course of your condition.

So how do you gain the confidence and skills to take an active part in managing your condition, communicate with health professionals and work through sometimes worrying and emotive issues? The answer is to become better informed. Reading about your problem, talking to others who have been through similar experiences and hearing what the experts have to say will all help to build-up your understanding and help you to take an active role in your own health care.

BESTMEDICINE Simple Guides provide an invaluable source of help, giving you the facts that you need in order to understand the key issues and discuss them with your doctors and other professionals involved in your care. The information is presented in an accessible way but without neglecting the important details. Produced independently and under the guidance of medical experts *A Simple Guide to Type 2 Diabetes* is an evidence-based, balanced and up-to-date review that I hope you will find enables you to play an active part in the successful management of your condition.

what happens normally?

WHAT HAPPENS NORMALLY?

In order to understand what's going on when you have type 2 diabetes, it is important to first understand what happens under normal circumstances.

IT'S ALL ABOUT SUGAR

A molecule is a group of atoms, and the smallest particle within a substance which shares its chemical properties.

Do you know what sugar is? 'Of course – it's the white crunchy stuff I sprinkle on my cornflakes.' But ask a scientist, and they will tell you that what we know of as sugar is, to give it its proper name, actually **sucrose**. Sucrose is a mixture of two smaller sugar molecules, called **glucose** and **fructose**. In fact, all carbohydrates that we eat are broken down during digestion to form glucose.

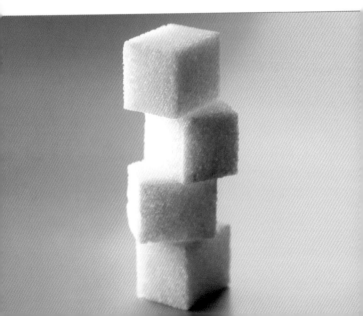

Glucose is the most important sugar as far as your body is concerned. This simple molecule is crucial for us to survive in good health, as it provides the link between the food we eat and the proper functioning of our bodies. The cells in our muscles, heart and brain, for example, get their energy from glucose. Essentially, glucose is the body's fuel.

Cells are the individual units that make up all tissues in the body, like the brain, liver, heart and muscles. The human body contains billions of them.

'BLOOD SUGAR' IS 'BLOOD GLUCOSE'

Your blood sugar level refers to the amount of glucose dissolved in your blood. Once glucose has been generated by the digestion of carbohydrates in the gut, it is then absorbed into the blood. Then, the glucose is taken around the body to tissues like the muscles, heart and brain, which can use it for energy.

Some glucose is taken to the liver, where it is stored in a slightly different form, called glycogen. This stored glucose can be released back into the blood as a 'back-up' between meals, when blood sugar levels fall.

If cells do not receive the glucose they need, they don't work properly. For this reason, blood sugar levels are kept within a tight range in a healthy person, to make sure that there is always enough glucose available for the cells which need it. But even if there is plenty of glucose in the blood, it is no use if it can't get into the cells. **This is where insulin comes in**.

The healthy range for 'fasting' blood sugar (not following a meal) is between 4 and 7 mmol/L. Two hours after a meal, blood sugar should be no higher than 9 mmol/L.

3

INSULIN IS THE KEY

In order for cells to be able to use the glucose that is in the blood to make energy, they need to be 'unlocked', and insulin is the key. Insulin is a hormone, made in the pancreas.

There is a steady release of insulin from beta-cells in the pancreas into the blood all the time. However, when blood sugar levels rise after a meal, there is a short burst of increased insulin released from the pancreas.

The pancreas is a tongue-shaped gland which sits below and behind the stomach.

Along with the glucose, insulin is then transported around the body in the blood to the cells which are in need of 'fuel'. On the surface of these cells are 'landing pads' for insulin, known as **receptors**. These receptors are a bit like tiny keyholes for the insulin 'key'. When insulin lands on one of these receptors, it 'unlocks' the cell, allowing glucose to get in.

When this system is working properly, blood sugar levels remain fairly constant throughout the day. When blood sugar rises, for example after a meal, the extra insulin that is released from the pancreas allows the

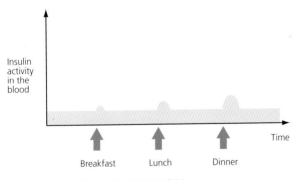

INSULIN RELEASE OVER THE COURSE OF A DAY.

FOUR STEPS TO BLOOD SUGAR CONTROL

1 Blood sugar level increases (e.g. after a meal).

2 More insulin released into blood.

3 More uptake of glucose into cells (e.g. liver, muscle, fatty tissue).

4 Blood sugar level falls.

glucose to be taken up into cells, restoring the level in the blood back to normal.

On the other hand, when insulin levels are low, the liver releases glucose from its glycogen stores to top up the blood sugar level.

Insulin allows the body to use glucose as its fuel.

INSULIN AND FATS

As well as controlling what happens to blood sugar, insulin also affects the way that the body uses fats. When blood sugar levels are low – between meals, for example – then the amount of insulin in the blood is also low. With the insulin signal – 'keep fat stores intact' – becoming weak, these stores are broken down, releasing **fatty acids** into the blood. These act as an alternative energy supply for when there is not enough glucose available.

Essentially, insulin 'keeps fats where they ought to be'.

5

When there are lots of fatty acids in the blood, the liver converts some of them into larger fatty substances, including cholesterol. All of these fat-like substances in the body are collectively known as **lipids**.

INSULIN IN CONTROL

- If you have eaten a meal recently, the **increased insulin** in your blood makes sure that the glucose released from the food gets into the cells, where it can be used to generate energy.
- If you haven't eaten recently, the **lack of insulin** in the blood acts as a signal to release glucose from glycogen stores in the liver, and to provide an alternative fuel (fatty acids) if glucose levels still fall too low.

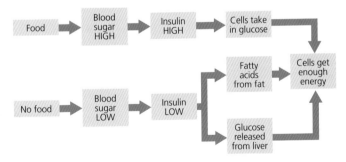

THE BASIC EFFECTS OF INSULIN.

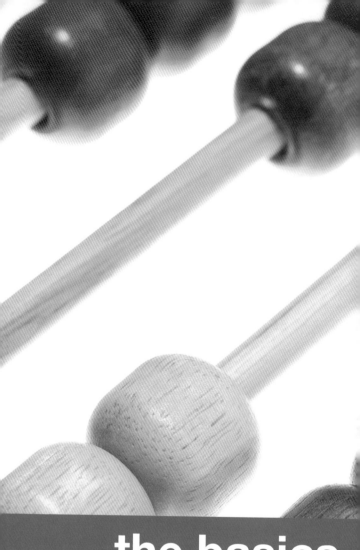

the basics

TYPE 2 DIABETES – THE BASICS

If you have diabetes, your insulin system does not work properly. The cells in your body cannot get enough glucose out of the blood because they remain 'locked' and so your blood sugar level is not controlled in the way it should be.

'Diabetes' is a Greek word meaning 'excessive urination'. 'Mellitus' is a Latin word meaning 'like honey'. If you have diabetes, your urine is sweet because your body is getting rid of sugar it cannot use.

The full name for diabetes is 'diabetes mellitus'. There are two main types of diabetes.

- In **type 1 diabetes**, the pancreas becomes damaged and stops producing insulin properly. In almost all cases, insulin production ceases completely. The problem usually starts in childhood, although some people develop type 1 diabetes when they are adults (a famous example being the Olympic rower, Sir Steven Redgrave – diagnosed at the age of 35).

- In **type 2 diabetes**, there are two problems. First, the cells in the body tissues become unable to respond properly (resistant) to insulin. This means that the pancreas has to work harder to produce more insulin. This causes the second problem: after a while, the cells in the pancreas become 'worn out' and are unable to produce insulin as effectively as they used to. This generally happens after the age of 40.

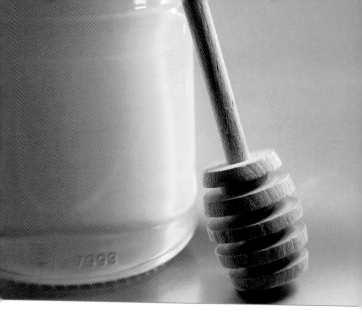

If you have type 1 diabetes, you need insulin treatment to survive, which explains why this form of the disease is also known as **'insulin-dependent diabetes mellitus (IDDM)'**. In type 2 diabetes, the pancreas still produces some of its own insulin, so this form of the disease has been referred to in the past as **'non-insulin-dependent diabetes mellitus (NIDDM)'**. This name is not very helpful though, as some people with type 2 diabetes are actually treated with insulin. It is much more acceptable these days just to refer to them as type 1 and 2. Type 2 diabetes is much more common than the type 1 form of the disease.

More than three-quarters of all people with diabetes in the UK have type 2 diabetes.

WHY IS TYPE 2 DIABETES A PROBLEM?

If you have type 2 diabetes, your cells are not getting enough glucose for two reasons:

■ your cells (particularly those in your muscles and fat stores) are resistant to insulin, and so are less likely to be 'unlocked' by it

■ there is less insulin in your blood.

Imagine the cells in your muscles (or other tissues) are covered in lots of tiny keyholes and insulin is the key that fits them.The diagram below illustrates what goes wrong in type 2 diabetes, using this lock and key analogy:

MUSCLE   **BLOOD**

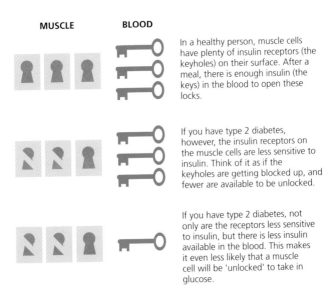

In a healthy person, muscle cells have plenty of insulin receptors (the keyholes) on their surface. After a meal, there is enough insulin (the keys) in the blood to open these locks.

If you have type 2 diabetes, however, the insulin receptors on the muscle cells are less sensitive to insulin. Think of it as if the keyholes are getting blocked up, and fewer are available to be unlocked.

If you have type 2 diabetes, not only are the receptors less sensitive to insulin, but there is less insulin available in the blood. This makes it even less likely that a muscle cell will be 'unlocked' to take in glucose.

THE LOCK AND KEY ANALOGY FOR DIABETES.

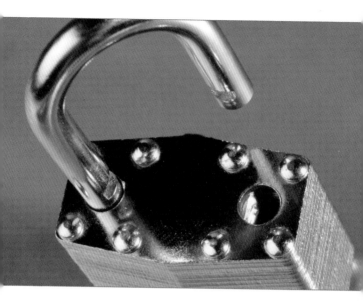

Because the cells in your muscles are taking in much less glucose, your blood sugar levels will remain high after a meal, instead of being brought back down to normal as they would be in a healthy person.

Despite the fact that there is plenty of glucose in your blood, your cells are not getting the amount of glucose that they should normally receive after a meal. Essentially, your cells do not recognise that you have eaten. Because of this, your body then sets about releasing glucose from other sources and alternative energy supplies, as it would in a healthy person who has not eaten for some time:

- the **liver** releases glucose into the blood from its glycogen stores
- stores of **fat** are broken down, releasing fatty acids into the blood.

If you have diabetes, your blood sugar levels will be abnormally high.

11

Your body's ongoing attempt to supply more glucose can also lead to muscles wasting and becoming weaker. If your body breaks down the proteins in muscle tissue, the liver can use the fragments to make glucose.

So, not only are your blood sugar levels high because the cells are not using up the glucose obtained from your diet, but they are increased even further because your body is releasing the 'back-up' supplies of glucose. And this is all because of your failing insulin system.

If you have type 2 diabetes, the lack of insulin in your blood after a meal causes fat stores to be broken down to release more glucose, when it is not actually needed. Not only does this increase blood sugar, but it also increases the levels of lipids (cholesterol and other fatty substances) in the blood. High blood lipid levels are responsible for increasing the risk of some of the complications of type 2 diabetes.

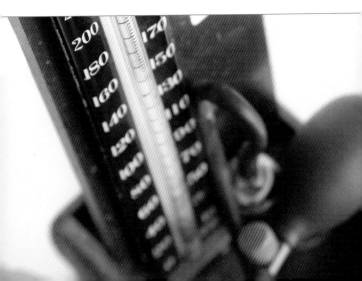

THE COMPLICATIONS OF TYPE 2 DIABETES

Type 2 diabetes can lead to some potentially serious complications, but the risks of these can be minimised if blood sugar levels are well controlled on a day-to-day basis.

The main complications which can result from type 2 diabetes are:

- coronary heart disease and stroke
- diabetic retinopathy (eye disease) and cataracts
- diabetic neuropathy (nerve damage)
- diabetic nephropathy (kidney disease).

If you are aware of these risks, you will recognise the importance of controlling your blood sugar levels and making full use of the team of professionals who are available to help you.

A linking factor between diabetes and some of these complications is high blood pressure, or hypertension. Having type 2 diabetes roughly doubles your risk of hypertension. Although hypertension does not directly cause any symptoms of its own, it can be very dangerous. Your diabetes management programme will include rigorous treatment to lower your blood pressure, if you are suffering from this problem.

THE SYMPTOMS OF TYPE 2 DIABETES

The excess glucose in the blood which is not used by cells is passed through the kidneys into the urine to be removed from the body. This may mean that you:

- need to urinate more often
- are often thirsty
- have more urinary infections (e.g. cystitis, thrush).

In type 2 diabetes your cells do not get enough glucose. Fat and protein stores are broken down to allow the glucose they contain to be released into the blood, but this can cause:

- unexplained weight loss
- tiredness.

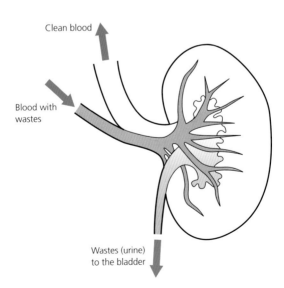

Clean blood

Blood with wastes

Wastes (urine) to the bladder

THE KIDNEY REMOVES WASTES (INCLUDING EXCESS GLUCOSE) FROM THE BLOOD.

Long periods of high blood sugar, high blood lipid levels and failed energy production can cause:

- blurred vision
- tingling, pain or ulceration in the feet
- frequent infections, especially thrush.

You need not be experiencing all of these symptoms to be diagnosed as having type 2 diabetes. They tend to emerge slowly, and you may have developed the disease some time before you experience any symptoms at all.

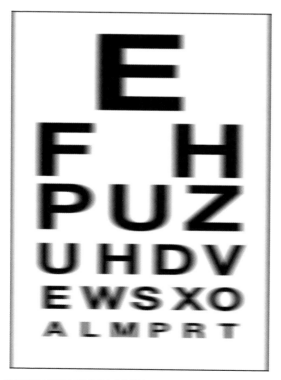

BLURRED VISION CAN BE A SYMPTOM OF TYPE 2 DIABETES.

THE CAUSES OF TYPE 2 DIABETES

The causes of type 2 diabetes are not completely understood. The major cause appears to be consuming too many calories compared to the amount being burnt off. Typically, if you have type 2 diabetes, the balance between the amount you eat and the amount of exercise you do will be tipped in the direction of over-eating.

Inheriting an increased risk of diabetes in your genes is the other main factor thought to cause type 2 diabetes. **Insulin resistance**, which is an essential step in the development of type 2 diabetes, can be triggered by an increase in body weight in people who are at increased risk because of a family history of diabetes.

Other factors which are thought to increase your risk of type 2 diabetes include:
- advancing age
- Afro-Caribbean or Asian ethnicity
- a previous history of 'gestational diabetes' (a form of diabetes which first occurs during pregnancy)
- a diagnosis of 'metabolic syndrome' (a collection of problems relating to the chemical reactions that go on inside the body).

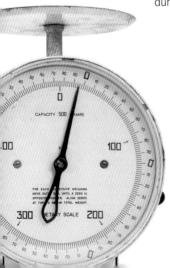

DIAGNOSING TYPE 2 DIABETES

If you are experiencing some of the symptoms described above, it is important that you visit your GP. In making a diagnosis, your GP may ask about your:

- symptoms
- family history
- eating and exercising habits
- weight
- age.

Although a urine test for glucose can offer a quick indication of whether or not you have diabetes, your doctor will test for the glucose content in your blood in order to offer you a definite diagnosis. If you have type 2 diabetes, this measurement will be abnormally high. The tests which might be done include:

- **random blood glucose** – on a blood sample taken at any time. A blood sugar level of at least 11.1 mmol/L indicates diabetes.
- **fasting blood glucose** – on a blood sample usually taken first thing in the morning, before you have had anything to eat (after an overnight 'fast'). A blood sugar level of at least 7 mmol/L indicates diabetes.
- **oral glucose tolerance test** – following an overnight fast, you will be given a sugary drink. A blood sample will be taken 10 minutes before and 2 hours after this drink. At the two-hour point, a blood sugar level of at least 11.1 mmol/L indicates diabetes.

MANAGING TYPE 2 DIABETES

Because type 2 diabetes is a long-term (or chronic) condition, it requires continuous management. If it is diagnosed early enough and managed properly, it may actually be possible to reverse some aspects of diabetes. Even in more severe cases, as long as your diabetes is managed properly:

- your blood sugar levels will be controlled
- your risk of developing long-term complications will be minimised
- you will be able to lead a normal, active life.

Once your type 2 diabetes has been diagnosed, you are likely to be supported by a care team of doctors, nurses, experts and, of course, your family. Because diabetes can cause a number of complications, this team may also include a chiropodist or an ophthalmologist.

Most people associate having diabetes with an absolute dependence on insulin injections. However, insulin injection is the least frequently used option of the three main strategies for managing type 2 diabetes:

- lifestyle modification
- antidiabetic tablets
- insulin injections.

FIVE IDEAS FOR AN ANTIDIABETIC LIFESTYLE

1. Cut down the total number of calories you consume each day.

2. Base your diet more on carbohydrates (e.g. bread, pasta, cereals, rice, potatoes) with less emphasis on proteins (e.g. meats, dairy produce) and fats (e.g. fatty meat, butter).

3. Aim for unsaturated rather than saturated fats (generally, vegetable-based fats such as olive oil, nuts and seeds as opposed to animal-based fats such as cheese, lard and suet).

4. Do more aerobic exercise, such as walking, running, playing sport or cycling.

5. If you smoke, stop!

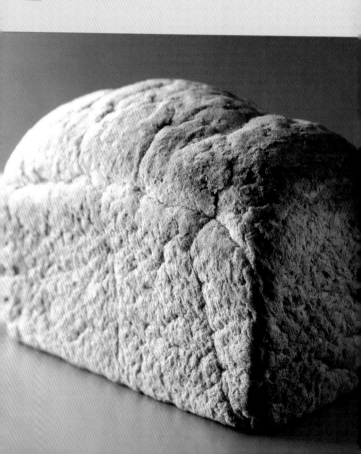

Your doctor will advise you to introduce more exercise into your lifestyle, and to ensure that you are eating a healthy, balanced diet.

If you make suitable lifestyle changes but your blood sugar level is still not adequately controlled, you may be prescribed antidiabetic tablets. There are five main groups of these drugs, all of which help to control blood sugar levels:

- **Biguanides** (e.g. metformin [Glucophage®, Glucophage SR®])
- **Sulphonylureas** (e.g. glibenclamide [Euglucon®], gliclazide [Diamicron®])
- **Prandial glucose regulators** (nateglinide [Starlix®], repaglinide [NovoNorm®])
- **Thiazolidinediones** (pioglitazone [Actos®], rosiglitazone [Avandia®])
- **Alpha glucosidase inhibitor** – (Acarbose [Glucobay®]).

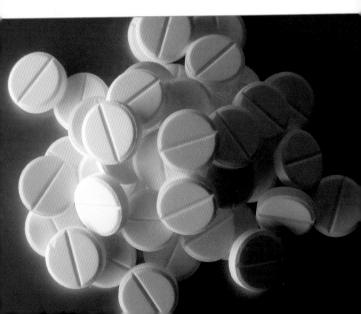

RECOGNISING HYPOGLYCAEMIA

There is a risk with some of these drugs that they can cause blood sugar levels to go too far the other way – they can fall dangerously low. This is called **hypoglycaemia**. If you experience mild hypoglycaemia, you can manage it without medical help, by consuming a sugary food or drink. However, if hypoglycaemia is moderate or severe, you will need help and possibly emergency treatment. It is important to know how to recognise hypoglycaemia before it gets too serious. Early signs may include:

- sweating
- hunger
- trembling
- headache
- becoming pale
- crying, temper, aggression
- rapid heart beat
- drowsiness, confusion.

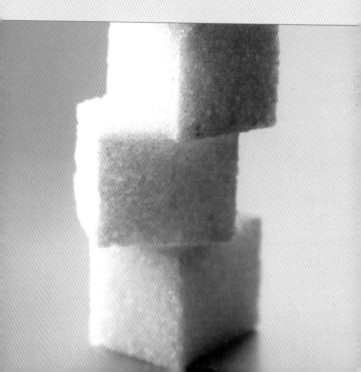

If your blood sugar level is not controlled with the combination of lifestyle changes and antidiabetic tablets, you may be asked to try insulin injections. Approximately 1 in 6 type 2 diabetes patients use insulin injections in the UK at the moment.

As you have seen, high blood pressure or 'hypertension' is common in people with type 2 diabetes. Your doctor will check your blood pressure regularly, and if it is high, you will probably be prescribed drugs to bring it down to normal levels.

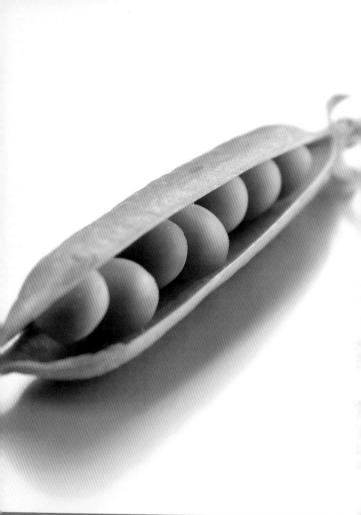

why me?

WHY ME?

If you, or a member of your family, have recently been diagnosed with diabetes, you're not alone. Type 2 diabetes is one of the most common chronic (long-term) diseases, currently affecting over 170 million people worldwide.

HOW COMMON IS TYPE 2 DIABETES?

If you, or a member of your family, have recently been diagnosed with type 2 diabetes, you're certainly not alone. Nearly 1.8 million people in the UK had diabetes (type 1 and 2) in 2000, and it is predicted that this figure will rise to over 2.5 million by the year 2030. In addition, there may be a further 1 million cases undiagnosed. Over three-quarters of all diabetes cases are type 2.

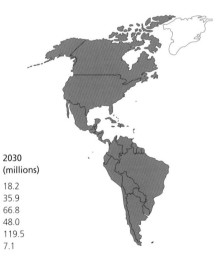

2000 (millions)	2030 (millions)
7.0	18.2
15.2	35.9
33.0	66.8
33.3	48.0
46.9	119.5
35.8	7.1

THE INCIDENCE OF DIABETES IN THE YEAR 2000, AND THE PREDICTED INCIDENCE IN 2030 (WHO).

CHANGING TRENDS IN DIABETES

The proportion of people being diagnosed with type 2 diabetes in the UK is rising steadily. The number of people with diabetes worldwide is expected to rise by more than one-third between 2000 and 2030. The most likely reason for this worrying trend is the increasing proportion of the population who are overweight and not doing enough exercise.

As we have seen, your risk of developing type 2 diabetes increases as you get older. Recent advances in medicine have helped people to live longer, and so this is also likely to lead to type 2 diabetes becoming more common.

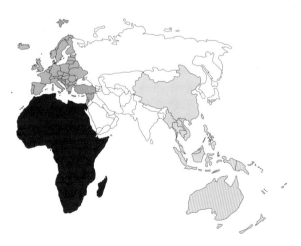

WHO GETS DIABETES?

Some people are more susceptible to developing type 2 diabetes than others. There are certain factors which make a person more likely to develop type 2 diabetes:

- being overweight
- not exercising enough
- a family history of diabetes
- advancing age
- high blood pressure and cholesterol levels
- having previously developed 'gestational diabetes' during pregnancy
- metabolic syndrome ('syndrome X')
- being of Asian or Afro-Caribbean ethnicity.

TYPE 2 DIABETES AND BODYWEIGHT

Probably the most established risk factor for developing type 2 diabetes is being overweight. Over 80% of people with type 2 diabetes are overweight, with a body mass index (BMI) of over 25. Overeating reduces the sensitivity of cells to insulin – an important factor in the development of type 2 diabetes. Calculate your BMI using the guidance overleaf.

Over the past 10 years, the number of obese 6-year-olds in the UK has doubled, and the number of obese 15-year-olds has trebled. In the same period, the number of children with type 2 diabetes has climbed from virtually none to roughly 1,400.

If your BMI indicates that you are overweight, you can get a better idea of your risk of type 2 diabetes (as well as other conditions such as heart disease) by looking at your body shape. Evidence suggests that it is very important where the fat is stored in your body. For example, you are more at risk of type 2 diabetes if your fat is stored around your waist (making you 'apple-shaped') than if it is mostly on your thighs and hips (making you 'pear-shaped'). Work out if you are an apple or a pear!

- Measure your waist and your hips in centimetres.
- Divide your waist measurement by your hip measurement.
- If the answer is greater than 1.0 (men) or 0.8 (women) you are 'apple-shaped'.

The fat that accumulates round your waist releases a protein which can make cells resistant to insulin. This is why being 'apple-shaped' increases your risk of type 2 diabetes.

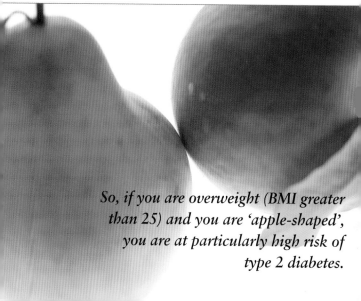

So, if you are overweight (BMI greater than 25) and you are 'apple-shaped', you are at particularly high risk of type 2 diabetes.

CALCULATE YOUR OWN BODY MASS INDEX (BMI)

It's very simple to work out your own BMI, to see whether your weight has put you at risk of type 2 diabetes. Grab a tape measure, a set of bathroom scales and a calculator and follow these two steps:

- Measure your height in metres. Multiply this number by itself and write down the answer.
- Measure your weight in kilograms. Divide it by the number you wrote down in the first step. *The number you get is your BMI.*

For example: if your height is 1.80 metres, when you multiply this by itself you get 3.24. If your weight is 80 kilograms, divide 80 by 3.24 to give 24.7.

As a general rule, for adults aged over 20:

	18.5	25	30	40
Underweight	Ideal weight	Overweight	Obese	Very obese

Remember though that your BMI is only a broad indicator – it is affected by your body style – people with a very muscular build will have a higher BMI but may not be unhealthily fat. Your age and gender also affect your BMI. Some experts say that men can have a slightly higher BMI before they are at risk, probably due to the fact that they are usually more muscular than women. However, it is best to stick to the guidelines above – they are the internationally accepted boundaries for both genders. The BMI scale does not apply to children though, or during pregnancy.

TYPE 2 DIABETES AND EXERCISE

Inadequate levels of exercise are closely associated with being overweight and result in a failure to burn off enough calories given the number consumed in the diet. A lack of exercise also makes you more likely to develop certain complications of diabetes, particularly heart disease.

Aerobic exercise is most important in diabetes. Activities which require short bursts of energy, such as sprinting or lifting weights, are not so useful, and may promote weight gain. They do not burn off as many calories as activities which require more stamina, such as walking, running, cycling, dancing or playing sports. Even cleaning and gardening can be good aerobic exercise!

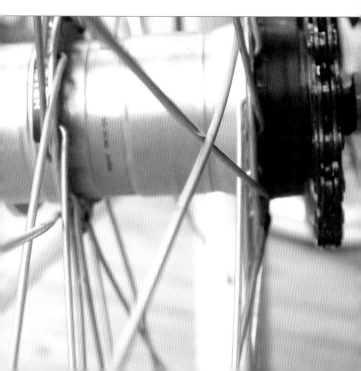

FAMILY HISTORY OF DIABETES

You can inherit an increased risk of type 2 diabetes in your genes.

If one of your parents, or a brother or sister, has diabetes, you are at a higher-than-average risk of developing type 2 diabetes yourself. The extent to which type 2 diabetes runs in families is greater than for type 1 diabetes. One study has shown that, of a sample of patients aged between 25 and 65 who had recently been diagnosed with type 2 diabetes, nearly half (41%) had a close relative with diabetes. It is thought to be virtually certain that if one of a pair of identical twins develops type 2 diabetes, the other will too. Although the evidence that type 2 diabetes can be inherited is very convincing, it is worth bearing in mind that families also tend to share similar lifestyles – for example, if a parent tends to eat excessively and does not exercise enough, it is likely that their children will adopt similar behaviour.

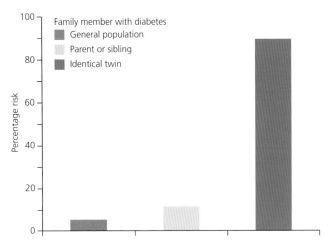

FAMILY RISK FOR TYPE 2 DIABETES.

TYPE 2 DIABETES AND AGE

Age is a strong risk factor for type 2 diabetes. Most people who develop type 2 diabetes are over the age of 45. Type 2 diabetes has been known in the past as 'late-onset' diabetes. However, as type 2 diabetes becomes more common, so do cases diagnosed in teenagers or even younger children.

The older you are, the more likely you are to develop diabetes.

This is most likely a reflection of the increased number of overweight and obese younger people in westernised countries. Nonetheless, it remains relatively rare in younger people – roughly 80% of all diabetes cases in the UK are type 2, but in the under-25-year age group, approximately 90% of cases are type 1. Younger people are most at risk of type 2 diabetes if they are overweight/obese, female, past puberty, of certain ethnicity (e.g. South Asian) and have a family history of diabetes.

A related condition is 'maturity onset diabetes of the young' (MODY), which generally occurs in patients under the age of 25. It is thought that 1–2% of all cases of diabetes might be MODY. The main problem in MODY is reduced insulin production by the pancreas, and it is treated in the same way as type 2 diabetes. However, MODY is not the same as type 1 or type 2 diabetes, and is passed on in families by means of a defective gene.

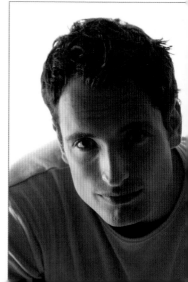

HIGH BLOOD PRESSURE AND CHOLESTEROL

Although type 2 diabetes increases the risk of getting high blood pressure and high blood cholesterol levels, these problems are also considered to be risk factors for type 2 diabetes. It is probably not so much a case of 'what causes what', but more the fact that these problems all share similar underlying causes. For example, being overweight can promote all three conditions – type 2 diabetes, high blood pressure and high cholesterol.

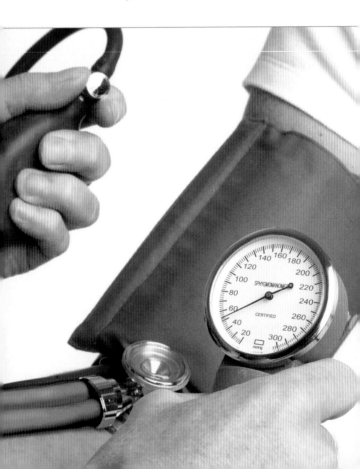

GESTATIONAL DIABETES

There is a form of diabetes which occurs in roughly 1 in 50 women during pregnancy, known as 'gestational diabetes'. If you have suffered from this in the past, or if you have previously given birth to a baby of over 10 pounds in weight (which suggests that you may have been experiencing gestational diabetes, whether you were aware of it or not), you have an increased risk of developing type 2 diabetes. Gestational diabetes can increase the risk of the baby developing type 2 diabetes or being overweight later in life.

TYPE 2 DIABETES AND METABOLIC SYNDROME

Metabolic syndrome, or 'syndrome X', is a collective term for a cluster of problems, including being overweight (particularly with an apple-shaped body), high blood pressure, high blood lipid levels and high insulin levels. If you have this condition, you are at increased risk of developing type 2 diabetes, as well as a range of other conditions such as heart disease and stroke.

TYPE 2 DIABETES AND ETHNIC ORIGIN

Your race is also important in determining your risk for type 2 diabetes. White (Caucasian) people are three-to-five times less likely to develop type 2 diabetes than people of Asian or Afro-Caribbean ethnicity. Type 2 diabetes also tends to develop at a younger age in these 'at-risk' groups.

DIABETES THROUGH HISTORY

1552 BC	The earliest known record of diabetes was written on Egyptian papyrus by the physician Hesy-Ra and listed frequent urination as a symptom.
First century AD	A Roman physician, Arateus, described diabetes as 'the melting down of flesh and limbs into urine'.
Second century	The Greek physician Galen of Pergamum mistakenly diagnosed diabetes as an ailment of the kidneys.
Up to the eleventh century	'Water tasters' were responsible for diagnosing diabetes. They had the unpleasant task of tasting the urine of people suspected of having diabetes, to assess its sweetness.
Early nineteenth century	Luckily for the water tasters, the first chemical tests were developed to detect and measure the levels of sugar in the urine.
1921	Insulin was officially 'discovered' in Canada, by the scientists Frederic Banting and Charles Best. The hormone was successfully used to treat a dog which had had its pancreas removed.
1922	The first human to be treated with insulin extract was a 14-year-old boy named Leonard Thompson. The treatment improved his condition within a few hours.
1940s	The link was established between diabetes and long-term complications such as diseases of the kidney and eye.

1955	The first oral drugs were introduced to lower blood sugar levels.
1959	The two distinct types of diabetes were first recognised: type 1 (insulin-dependent) and type 2 (non-insulin-dependent) diabetes.
1998	The UK Prospective Diabetes Study was published. The results of this 20-year study of over 5,000 patients clearly indicated the importance of good glucose and blood pressure control in the prevention or delay of the complications of type 2 diabetes.

THE LONG-TERM RISKS ASSOCIATED WITH TYPE 2 DIABETES

Type 2 diabetes itself may not seem to be causing you many problems, and you may wonder why there is such emphasis on making sure that it is well controlled. The longer you have type 2 diabetes, the higher your risk of developing complications. If your blood sugar, and hence your diabetes, is poorly controlled, these complications can begin to occur at an earlier age.

Coronary heart disease and stroke

Problems with the heart and blood vessels (cardiovascular disease) account for up to half of all deaths in the UK. However, approximately three-quarters of deaths are attributable to cardiovascular disease amongst people with diabetes, so there is clearly an

Nearly three-quarters of people with type 2 diabetes in the UK are unaware that their condition is linked with an increased risk of cardiovascular disease.

35

increased risk. By looking at the most important risk factors for cardiovascular disease, we can see that there is a considerable overlap between its causes and those of type 2 diabetes:

- high blood sugar
- high blood lipid levels
- high blood pressure
- smoking
- excess body weight.

Diabetic retinopathy (eye disease) and cataracts

Over a third of patients with type 2 diabetes are found to already have retinopathy when they are diagnosed, although only 1 in 20 of these cases is serious enough to be sight-threatening. If, however, there is no evidence of retinopathy at the stage of diagnosis, there is a much smaller risk (less than 1 in 100) of developing sight-threatening retinopathy within 2 years.

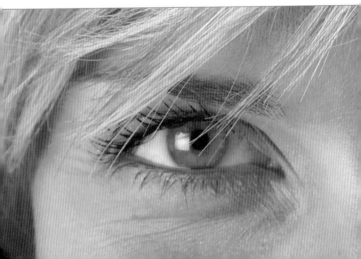

If you have diabetes, your risk of developing a cataract is roughly doubled compared with a healthy person. This risk is increased further if your blood sugar level is not properly controlled. With good day-to-day control of diabetes, however, the vast majority of patients with type 2 diabetes can avoid any loss of sight.

Diabetic neuropathy (nerve damage)

Between 20 and 40% of people with diabetes will develop diabetic neuropathy. By far the most common manifestations of diabetic neuropathy are problems with the feet. Roughly 1 in 20 people with diabetes will experience foot ulceration. It has been proven that awareness about the risks of foot disease can reduce the risks of developing serious problems, as thorough foot care can prevent or delay the effects of neuropathy.

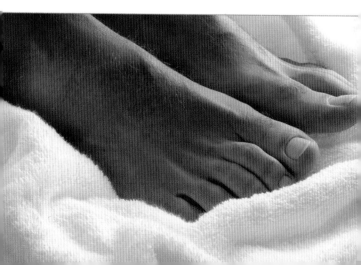

Diabetic nephropathy (kidney disease)

The mildest form of diabetic nephropathy is called **microalbuminuria**. Up to one-quarter of patients who have type 2 diabetes for 10 years will develop microalbuminuria in that time.

Of those who do develop microalbuminuria, approximately one-fifth will progress to the next stage of severity of nephropathy, **proteinuria**. This form of nephropathy can be very dangerous – only half of patients with proteinuria can live with the condition for more than 4 years.

Nephropathy is more common in men with diabetes than women, and is associated with high blood pressure. Good control of blood sugar and blood pressure are crucial in minimising the risk of this condition.

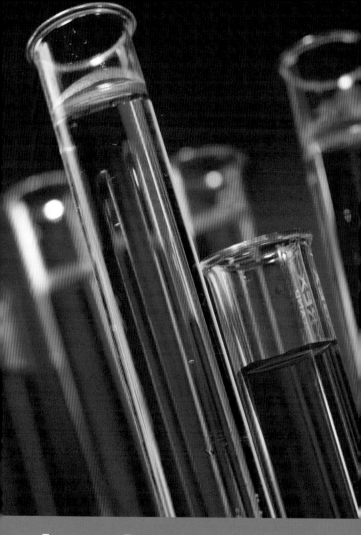

simple science

SIMPLE SCIENCE

In order for you to understand how the different treatments for type 2 diabetes work, you need to learn a little more about what goes wrong in type 2 diabetes.

We don't know exactly what causes insulin resistance. You can inherit an increased risk for insulin resistance, but excessive consumption of calories is thought to be another major contributing factor.

Type 2 diabetes is a combination of two main problems. Lots of people develop a resistance to the effects of insulin in their muscles, liver and fat stores, for example (like the blocking up of the cells' 'keyholes'). Roughly a quarter of the healthy population may be insulin resistant and not suffer any obvious ill effects. It is a particularly common feature in people with high blood pressure and heart disease.

About a third of people with insulin resistance go on to develop type 2 diabetes. Normally, a person with insulin resistance would simply produce more insulin to overcome the problem. However, in some people, the beta-cells of the pancreas stop working properly, and so insulin levels fall (like the reduced number of insulin 'keys'). Therefore, the combination of insulin resistance and reduced production of insulin is what causes type 2 diabetes.

ONE-IN-THREE PEOPLE WITH INSULIN RESISTANCE GO ON
TO DEVELOP TYPE 2 DIABETES.

The diagram opposite shows the main actions of insulin in a healthy person following a meal. It's all a case of which processes insulin kicks into action, and which ones it puts the brakes on. The pale sections in the diagram show processes that are 'put on hold' following a meal, whereas the darker sections are the processes that are activated. Follow the diagram through with this explanation:

- The carbohydrates from the meal are broken down into glucose in the gut, and the glucose absorbed from the gut into the blood increases blood sugar levels.
- The beta-cells of the pancreas respond to this increase in blood sugar by producing more insulin.
- This insulin stimulates cells in the muscles to take up and use the glucose to make energy. **This reduces blood sugar levels.**
- The insulin prevents the liver from releasing glucose from its stores into the blood. **Blood sugar levels are not increased.**
- The insulin prevents the fat stores from being broken down to release lipids into the blood. **The lipid content of the blood remains low.**

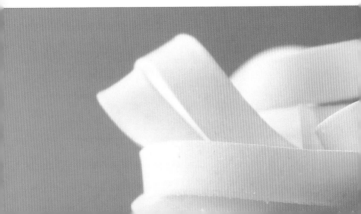

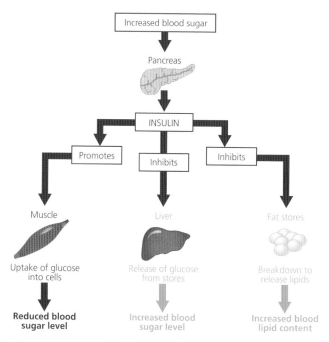

| Increased blood sugar |
| Pancreas |
| INSULIN |
Promotes	Inhibits	Inhibits
Muscle	Liver	Fat stores
Uptake of glucose into cells	Release of glucose from stores	Breakdown to release lipids
Reduced blood sugar level	Increased blood sugar level	Increased blood lipid content

THE ACTIONS OF INSULIN IN A HEALTHY PERSON FOLLOWING A MEAL.

Blood sugar levels are brought back down
to normal levels by insulin following the meal.
The cells in the muscles, as well as other tissues,
have taken up the glucose they need and fat
has stayed 'where it belongs', in the fat stores.

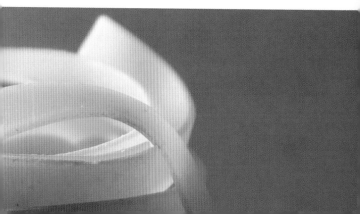

The next diagram shows how the situation changes if you have type 2 diabetes. The red arrows show the two points in the system where type 2 diabetes makes things go wrong.

- First, the beta-cells of the pancreas do not respond properly to the rise in blood sugar levels, and produce very little insulin.
- Secondly, cells in the muscle, liver and fat stores are resistant to the little insulin that is available.

Essentially, the body is acting as it would in a healthy person who had not just eaten – the cells are 'seeing' very little insulin in the blood, as if blood sugar had not increased.

- Therefore, muscle cells do not take up much glucose from the blood. **Blood sugar levels remain high.**
- The liver releases glucose from its stores into the blood, as it would between mealtimes in a healthy person. **Blood sugar levels increase further.**
- The fat stores are broken down to release lipids into the blood. **The lipid content of the blood increases.**

Therefore, if you have diabetes, a meal which is rich in carbohydrates causes your blood sugar level to increase out of control.

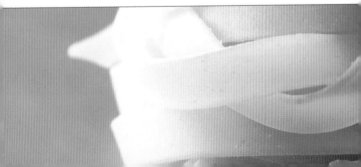

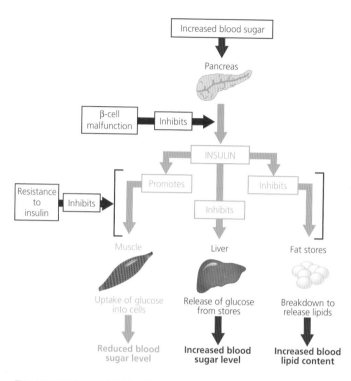

THE ACTIONS OF INSULIN IN A PERSON WITH TYPE 2 DIABETES.

Not only is your blood high in glucose, but it also now contains lots of lipids. This means that type 2 diabetes causes two main problems:

■ high blood sugar (technically called hyperglycaemia)
■ high levels of lipids in the blood (technically called hyperlipidaemia).

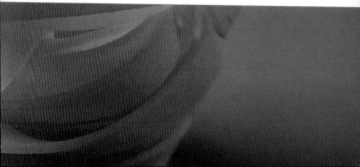

A third factor, which is not a direct consequence of diabetes, but is very closely related, is high blood pressure, or hypertension. As you have already seen, roughly half of people with diabetes also have hypertension. The reason for this close association is not entirely clear, but experts generally agree that the two conditions have overlapping causes. For example, an excessive amount of the fat which accumulates around the waist (leading to the 'apple-shape' that you read about earlier) is thought to affect blood vessels, making them more stiff. This can increase blood pressure, that is, cause hypertension.

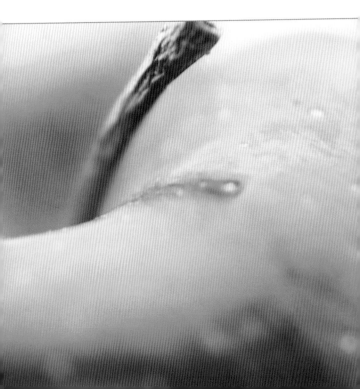

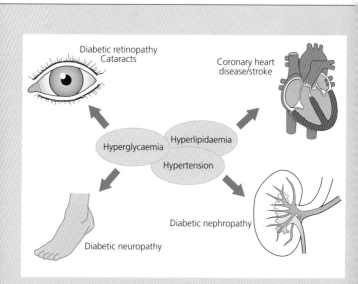

The combination of hyperglycaemia, hyperlipidaemia and, if you have it, hypertension can increase your risk of experiencing the complications of type 2 diabetes. Good management of your condition will target all three of these problems and help to reduce the risk of all of the complications.

THE METABOLIC SYNDROME

You are at increased risk of type 2 diabetes if you have **metabolic syndrome**, also known by a variety of other names including 'syndrome X', 'insulin resistance syndrome' and 'the deadly quartet'. This is a group of symptoms arising from problems with your metabolism (the chemical processes that naturally occur inside your body). Metabolic syndrome affects approximately one-quarter of the UK population. It is strongly linked with obesity and lack of exercise, and a family history of the syndrome also appears to increase the risk.

The 'deadly quartet' of related problems is:

- obesity (specifically the 'apple-shaped' abdominal obesity)
- hypertension
- hyperlipidaemia
- hyperinsulinaemia – excess insulin in the blood.

Blood sugar levels are high in metabolic syndrome, but not as high as in full-blown type 2 diabetes. The most important diagnostic criterion for metabolic syndrome is waist measurement. In order to be diagnosed with metabolic syndrome, your waist must be at least 94 cm (if you are a man) or 80 cm (if you are a woman). These

HOW DO ANTIDIABETIC DRUGS WORK?

The tablets that your doctor might prescribe you to control your diabetes are designed to bring your blood sugar level back down to what it should be. There are a number of different classes of these drugs, each of which works differently to bring blood sugar down.

values are relevant to a Caucasian person living in the UK, but the threshold varies with ethnicity.

You will notice that there are very close similarities between the causes and symptoms of metabolic syndrome with those of type 2 diabetes. Experts think that the same problem is responsible for both conditions – **insulin resistance**. In metabolic syndrome, the pancreas is able to compensate for the insulin resistance by producing more insulin, which explains the excess insulin in the blood or hyperinsulinaemia. However, if the pancreas cannot maintain this excessive rate of insulin production, the metabolic syndrome evolves into type 2 diabetes. The early stages of this transition are called **prediabetes**. If you have prediabetes, the beta-cells in your pancreas are beginning to fail and therefore insulin production is falling.

Obesity is a key factor in both metabolic syndrome and type 2 diabetes. Being overweight and inactive promotes insulin resistance in the first place. But remember that insulin resistance is reversible. Losing weight and doing more exercise can restore your cells' sensitivity to the effects of insulin, which takes the strain off your pancreas. This is crucial if you have metabolic syndrome, and want to reduce your risk of developing type 2 diabetes.

Biguanides

There is only one biguanide drug available in the UK – metformin (Glucophage®, Glucophage SR®). This drug reduces blood sugar levels through three main actions:

- it slows down the absorption of glucose from the gut into the blood
- it reduces the release of glucose from liver glycogen stores
- it increases the sensitivity of muscle cells to insulin.

Metformin makes the surge of blood sugar you experience after a meal more gradual and sustained. This makes it easier for your weak insulin system to deal with the extra glucose. On top of this, the liver continues to store glucose as glycogen, as it should do after a meal. The muscle cells also respond better to the little insulin that is available, so they take up glucose from the blood. In other words, when you are taking metformin, your body responds more normally to receiving a meal. Metformin has also been shown to reduce levels of lipids and cholesterol in the blood, suggesting that it inhibits the breakdown of fat stores that normally happens in type 2 diabetes.

Sulphonylureas

These drugs, which include glimepiride (Amaryl®) and gliclazide (Diamicron®), act by increasing the amount of insulin that the beta-cells produce, so directly addressing one of the two main causes of type 2 diabetes. They do not affect the sensitivity of cells to the effects of insulin. Because there is more insulin in the blood, however, more glucose is taken up into the muscles, less is released from the liver and fat stores remain intact. As a result, blood sugar and lipid levels fall.

Prandial glucose regulators

These drugs, of which nateglinide (Starlix®) and repaglinide (NovoNorm®) are the only two available in the UK, act in the same way as the sulphonylureas – they stimulate the beta-cells in the pancreas to produce more insulin. However, this effect does not last as long as it does with sulphonylureas, which means there is a slightly lower risk of hypoglycaemia.

Thiazolidinediones (glitazones)

These drugs, of which pioglitazone (Actos®) and rosiglitazone (Avandia®) are the only two available in the UK, act by increasing the sensitivity of cells in the muscle, fatty tissue and liver to the effects of insulin. In contrast to the sulphonylureas, they do not affect the amount of insulin being produced by the beta-cells in the pancreas.

Alpha glucosidase inhibitors

The only one of these drugs available in the UK is acarbose (Glucobay®). It inhibits an enzyme involved in the digestion of carbohydrates (called alpha-glucosidase), and in so doing, slows down the absorption of glucose into the blood.

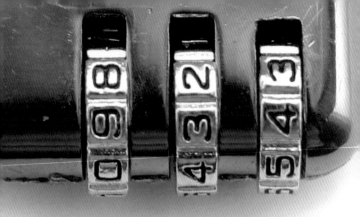

These drugs act by reducing blood sugar levels. Some of them carry a risk of 'overshooting' the safe limits, causing blood sugar levels to fall dangerously low (technically called hypoglycaemia).

In up to a quarter of patients treated with antidiabetic drugs, blood sugar will still not be adequately controlled, and the doctor will advise treatment with insulin injections. These injections, if you receive them, will of course raise your blood level of insulin. They will not, however, change the fact that the cells in the muscles and fatty tissue, for example, remain resistant to its effects.

In some patients, it may be appropriate to combine insulin treatment with antidiabetic drugs. The combination of insulin and metformin, for example, would be expected both to increase the level of insulin in the blood (due to the insulin injections) and increase the sensitivity of some cells to that insulin (due to the actions of metformin).

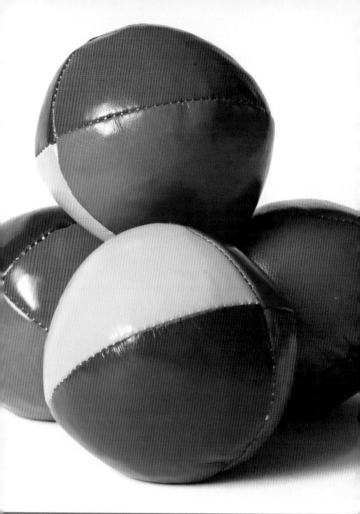

managing
type 2 diabetes

MANAGING TYPE 2 DIABETES

In order to minimise the effect that your type 2 diabetes has on your life, and the risk of long-term complications, you and your care team need to work together.

WHAT IS GOING TO HAPPEN TO ME?

You can lead a perfectly normal life with type 2 diabetes, and you will not be left to deal with it on your own.

Whether you have recently been diagnosed with type 2 diabetes or have been living with the condition for years, it is in your best interests to gain an understanding of what having diabetes means, and what the options are for treating it. This way, you can take an active role in the management of your condition, and understand the reasoning behind the advice you are given.

You will also be able to find further information through the various national and international support groups. Diabetes UK, for example, is an independent organisation providing information and support for people living with diabetes in the UK (*www.diabetes.org.uk*). Further organisations that offer help and advice are listed in the Simple Extras section.

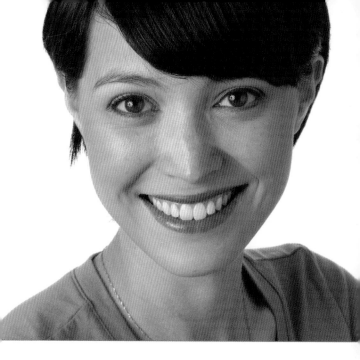

DIAGNOSIS

Your GP will be able to diagnose type 2 diabetes. At your first consultation, your doctor will listen to the symptoms you describe to him. Remember that the symptoms of type 2 diabetes come on gradually, and it is possible that you will have had the disease for some time before you started noticing them.

Your doctor will use blood tests to diagnose type 2 diabetes. There are three types of blood test which can be used to measure your blood sugar levels:

- random blood glucose test
- fasting blood glucose test
- oral glucose tolerance test.

Diabetes will be diagnosed if:

■ two consecutive fasting blood glucose tests give a result of at least 7 mmol/L (regardless of symptoms)

■ two consecutive random blood glucose tests give a result of at least 11.1 mmol/L (regardless of symptoms)

■ a random blood glucose test gives a result of at least 11.1 mmol/L and there are symptoms.

If you have prediabetes, you have roughly a one-in-twenty risk of going on to develop type 2 diabetes.

If the fasting or random blood glucose tests indicate that blood sugar is higher than normal, but not as high as the thresholds given above (in other words, in the ranges 6.1–7 mmol/L and 7.8–11.1 mmol/L, respectively), your doctor may use the oral glucose tolerance test to diagnose 'impaired glucose tolerance'. In this condition, also known as prediabetes, the beta-cells in your pancreas are just starting to fail. Your body is slow to deal with surges in blood sugar levels, but your insulin system is not as damaged as it would be in type 2 diabetes.

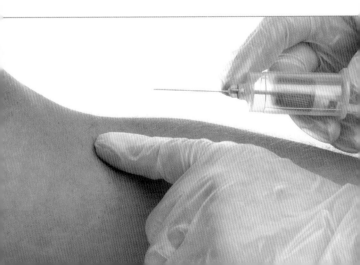

HOW CAN I BE SURE THAT I HAVE TYPE 2 AND NOT TYPE 1 DIABETES?

A number of factors will help your doctor to identify that you have type 2, rather than type 1 diabetes.

- **Age** – if you are first diagnosed over the age of 45, it is highly likely that you have type 2 diabetes.
- **Weight** – if your diabetes were type 1, you would be unlikely to be overweight.
- **Symptoms** – if these have come on gradually, it is likely that your diabetes is type 2.
- **Diabetic ketoacidosis** – if you experience an episode of this serious condition, it is unlikely that you have type 2 diabetes. It can cause loss of consciousness and can even be fatal, but generally only occurs in type 1 diabetes.
- **Family history** – in most cases of type 2 diabetes there is some family history. A lack of family history is more consistent with a diagnosis of type 1 diabetes.

YOUR DIABETES MANAGEMENT PLAN

Following your diagnosis, your doctor will give you a full medical examination, and then work with you to devise a suitable programme of care. This will include management goals, which are tailored to you and your lifestyle. If you are a younger person with type 2 diabetes, these goals are likely to be more demanding, since your risk of long-term complications increases the longer you have the disease.

In a broad sense, your management programme will aim to:

- control your everyday symptoms, allowing you to lead a normal life
- minimise your risk of long-term complications.

YOUR DIABETES CARE TEAM

The number of people involved in your 'care team' will depend on the severity of your type 2 diabetes, and whether you are affected by any complications. Here, we will look at a few of the main players.

Your GP

Your GP will provide you with the initial diagnosis of type 2 diabetes, and is responsible for introducing you to many of the other members of the care team who will co-ordinate your care. Together with the rest of the team, your GP will work with you to generate a programme of care. You will be invited for a check-up with your GP at least once a year, at which they may check your:

- blood pressure
- blood lipid levels
- HbA_{1c}
- kidney function
- urine, for protein content
- eyes for signs of retinopathy
- BMI
- feet, for signs of neuropathy.

Practice/diabetes specialist nurse

A nurse will offer information and advice on managing your diabetes. He/she might be responsible for running diabetic clinics, which you should attend every few months for regular checks and screening for complications.

Consultant diabetologist

This is the most specialised doctor in charge of diabetes care. Your GP may refer you to a consultant if:

- your diabetes is proving difficult to control
- you are experiencing new or worsening complications
- you are pregnant
- you are a particularly young type 2 diabetes patient.

THE HBA$_{1C}$ TEST

The HbA$_{1C}$ (sometimes referred to as just HbA$_1$) test gives a more long-term measurement of your blood sugar level than the fasting or random blood glucose tests used at diagnosis. The term HbA$_{1C}$ refers to glucose which is bound to haemoglobin, the component of your red blood cells responsible for carrying oxygen. The amount of haemoglobin in the blood which is bound to glucose is a direct reflection of the blood sugar level, so it can be used as a marker for glucose control.

You will need to provide a full blood sample, which will be sent off to a laboratory for the test to be performed. The results of the test provide an average of the blood sugar level over the last 2–3 months, because this is the life-span of a red blood cell. This test gives a very good indication of how well the diabetes is being controlled (control is good if the HbA$_{1C}$ result is less than 7%).

YOU

Always remember that you hold much of the responsibility for making sure that your diabetes is managed properly.

■ Take as much control as you can over managing your own condition. The more you learn about type 2 diabetes, the easier this will be. Reading this book is a very good start!

■ Take an active role in the management programme which your doctor devises for you.

■ Learn to monitor your own blood sugar levels, if your doctor recommends that you do so.

■ Know your limits – know what is normal (in terms of blood sugar levels and symptoms) and what should trigger you to ask for help.

■ Know how to contact members of your team when you need them.

■ Take the advice of other members of your team, and do your best to work it into your lifestyle.

■ Be aware of the potential complications of type 2 diabetes, and look out for early warning signs.

■ Always attend the appointments you are given.

■ Inform the relevant organisations (e.g. Driver and Vehicle Licensing Agency [DVLA]), of your condition if you are advised by a member of your team to do so.

MONITORING YOUR OWN BLOOD SUGAR LEVELS

Your doctor or nurse will be keeping an eye on your blood sugar levels. They will carry out HbA_{1c} tests at regular intervals to make sure that your blood sugar remains at a safe level. If your type 2 diabetes is being managed by lifestyle changes alone, or lifestyle changes with antidiabetic tablets, your doctor probably won't insist that you learn how to monitor your blood sugar levels at home. However, you may find it reassuring to do so, particularly if you are ill, as this may affect your blood sugar control. If you are receiving insulin treatment, it is recommended that you learn how to monitor your own blood sugar, and incorporate it into your self-management programme.

At home, you would measure your blood sugar level using a single drop blood test (usually from the side of a finger, near the fingertip). You need to put a single drop of your blood onto a test strip. You then place the strip in a meter, which will display the result in 5–20 seconds. Your blood sugar is uncontrolled if it is:

- over 7 mmol/L following an overnight fast
- over 11.1 mmol/L at any time.

You can buy a **glucose testing meter** for this purpose from most chemists, or your diabetes clinic may be able to supply you one on loan. Your practice/diabetes nurse will be able to demonstrate how to use the meter properly. Glucose testing meters available in the UK include the Accutrend® and Glucometer® GX/4.

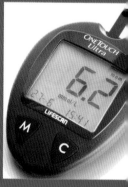

Always remember to wash your hands before taking a blood drop sample for a home blood glucose test, otherwise you may contaminate the strip with sugar from your fingers.

LIFESTYLE MODIFICATION

The first thing that your GP will ask you to do in order to improve your condition is to modify your lifestyle. This might conjure up images in your head of a restrictive diabetic diet and constant monitoring of blood sugar levels. Don't panic – the changes you will need to make are positive ones! You may also feel like you are being blamed for having your condition. There is no need to feel like this. Although your lifestyle will have contributed to your development of type 2 diabetes, not everyone who has a diabetogenic lifestyle develops the condition.

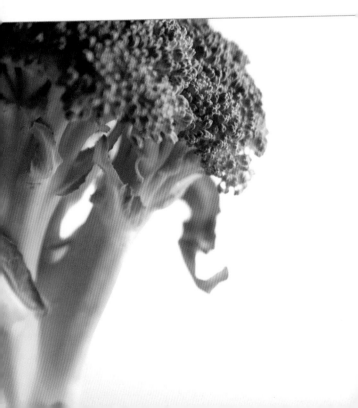

You also shouldn't feel that your doctor is trivialising your condition by advising you to modify your lifestyle. If you are overweight, the UK guidelines which doctors follow (the National Institute for Health and Clinical Excellence [NICE] guidelines) do not recommend the use of drugs until it is clear to them that, despite your best attempts to improve your lifestyle, your blood sugar levels have not been brought under control. If you can get your condition under control without the need for drugs, this is best for you, as the drugs have a range of side-effects, including a risk of causing dangerously low blood sugar levels.

A HEALTHY DIET

Not everyone with type 2 diabetes is overweight. Every type 2 diabetes patient can benefit from a healthy diet, though! Your GP may introduce you to a dietitian, who will be able to advise you on how to modify your diet. There is no reason for you to buy expensive special diabetic foods. These tend to be just as high in calorie and fat content as normal foods, and some of the sweeteners included can have laxative effects. The healthy diet that you should follow is the same as that recommended for people who do not have diabetes. Your diet should:

- be rich in starchy foods, such as bread, pasta, potatoes, cereals and rice
- be low in fat, sugar and salt
- include plenty of fruits and vegetables.

The UK government's Food Standards Agency (*www.food.gov.uk*) has produced a picture food guide called *The Balance of Good Health*, which shows in what proportions you should aim to eat the five main food groups:

- bread, cereals and potatoes
- fruit and vegetables
- milk and dairy foods
- meat, fish and alternatives
- fatty and sugary foods.

The size of the section on the plate taken up by each type of food represents what proportion of your diet it should make up.

'THE BALANCE OF GOOD HEALTH'.

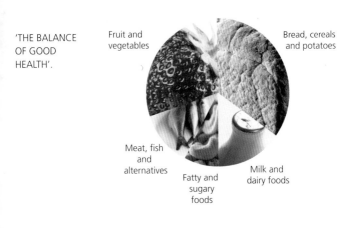

Fruit and vegetables

Bread, cereals and potatoes

Meat, fish and alternatives

Fatty and sugary foods

Milk and dairy foods

In order to model your diet on *The Balance of Good Health*, you will need to:

- eat regular meals, at similar times each day
- base your meals on starchy foods such as bread, pasta, rice, potatoes and cereals
- make sure there is plenty of fibre in your diet

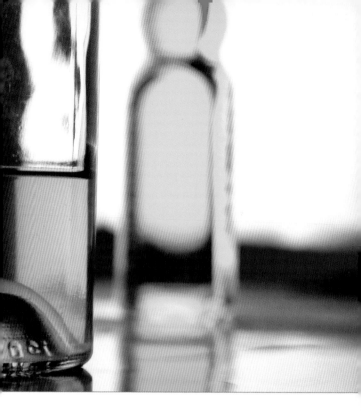

- cut down on the amount of fatty foods you eat – try to choose monounsaturated fats such as olive and rapeseed oil, and opt for low fat varieties of dairy foods (e.g. skimmed milk and low fat yoghurt)
- eat more fruit and vegetables – try to eat at least five portions per day
- choose low sugar versions of sugary foods and drinks – you need not cut out sugar altogether, but try to limit the amount you eat
- use less salt – be aware of the salt content in the foods you eat – it is often higher than you might expect.

Aside from these general guidelines, you may wish to try and use specific dietary concepts to establish whether they help with your blood sugar control. You should not embark on one of these strategies without first talking it through with your GP or dietitian, as it is important to integrate your diet into your complete care programme. If your doctor advises that the diet you intend to follow is not advisable for you personally, listen to them and respect their expertise.

THE 'LOW GI' DIET

The sugar you put on your cornflakes actually has a lower GI value than the cornflakes themselves!

The Glycaemic Index, or GI, is a ranking system for foods which contain carbohydrates based on how they affect your blood sugar levels.

■ **Low GI foods** are absorbed slowly, causing a slow, sustained increase in blood sugar.
■ **High GI foods** are absorbed quickly, causing a rapid and sizeable increase in blood sugar.

Glucose is taken as the 'reference' food, with a GI rating of 100. Foods being tested against this reference contain the same total amount of carbohydrate as the glucose sample, in order to make it a fair comparison.

From the point of view of gaining good control of your blood sugar through your diet, a good rule of thumb is to aim for foods with low GI values. Your ailing insulin system will find it easier to cope with low GI foods, and your blood sugar should remain more stable.

Low GI (under 55)	Medium GI (56–69)	High GI (70 or more)
Milk	Sucrose	Jelly beans
Apples, pears, oranges, peaches, grapes, bananas, grapefruit, kiwi	Raisins, sultanas	Parsnips (boiled)
All Bran	Fresh pineapple/melon	White rice (steamed)
Orange/apple juice	Mars Bar	Swede
Baked beans	Ryvita	Bagel
Milk chocolate	Wholemeal bread	White bread
Peanuts (salted/roasted)	Digestive biscuit	Cornflakes, branflakes

There is no need to cut out all high GI foods. Simply try to use foods with low GI values to bring down the average GI rating for each meal you eat.

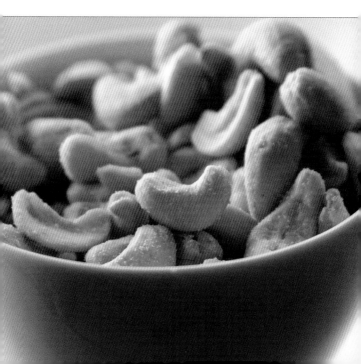

THE 'LOW-CARB' DIET

This one is a little more controversial. Standard guidelines advise you to base your diet mainly on carbohydrates, with a much smaller contribution from fats. However, there is a growing school of thought which suggests that excessive consumption of carbohydrates is, in fact, the root of the problem, causing obesity, type 2 diabetes and numerous other health problems.

Low-carb diets involve a considerable restriction of the amount of carbohydrates in the diet, with calories instead obtained mostly from fats, meats, eggs and small amounts of salad. It may not seem very intuitive given the greater amount of fat in the diet, but there is good evidence that this approach can help with weight-loss programmes.

This is the rationale behind the controversial Atkins diet, and is subject to a lot of controversy and safety fears, especially concerning the risk of heart disease. However, support is growing for the adoption of a modified Atkins style of diet for type 2 diabetic patients. If you are tempted to try a low-carb diet, it is vital that you discuss it with your doctor first. It is not advisable if you are receiving insulin injections, and contravenes the more recognised diet advice for people with type 2 diabetes.

EGGS FORM PART
OF A 'LOW-CARB'
DIET.

LOSING WEIGHT

If you are overweight, like 80% of all people with type 2 diabetes, it is important that you try to lose weight. Obesity makes your body less sensitive to insulin, so losing weight will have an antidiabetic effect, and help to control your blood sugar and reduce your risk of long-term complications.

You should aim to lose weight gradually, and following *The Balance of Good Health* model will help you to do this. As well as eating the different food types in the correct proportions, it is also important that you don't eat too much. There are recommended daily limits to how many calories and how much fat you should include in your diet each day, and if you stick to these limits, this will help in achieving a healthy weight.

Work together with your GP or dietitian to develop a sensible weight-loss plan. Don't aim for an over-ambitious 'quick fix'. If you approach it sensibly, and set realistic goals, you are much more likely to keep the weight off in the long-term.

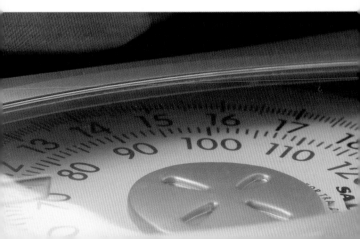

RECOMMENDED DAILY ALLOWANCES FOR THE AVERAGE ADULT		
Each day	Women	Men
Calories	2000	2500
Fat	70 g (saturates 20 g)	95 g (saturates 30 g)

- ■ Try not to skip meals – eat regular meals to avoid hunger pangs which make you snack!

- ■ Enjoy your food – eating more slowly fills you up more, so you won't feel the need to eat as much.

- ■ Only weigh yourself once a week – if you weigh yourself every day, you will only get disheartened by the ups and downs in your weight that occur naturally.

- ■ Give yourself plenty of variety – look out for low-calorie, low-fat recipes and try new things.

- ■ Eat plenty of foods which are high in fibre – these will satisfy your hunger.

- ■ Remember that alcohol contains more calories than you might expect.

- ■ Join a slimming group – the support of other people will help you to stick to a weight-loss plan.

EATING FATS

Although you are trying to lose weight, do not aim to cut out fats altogether. Your diet needs to be balanced and fats are needed for your body to function properly. They are a crucial component of the structure of all the cells in your body, and there are vitamins that are only soluble in fat. It is even thought by some experts that very low fat diets can aggravate type 2 diabetes.

Where fats are concerned, aim to:
- keep within your total recommended daily allowance
- choose unsaturated fats (monounsaturated and polyunsaturated) in preference to saturated fats.

Saturated fats lead to increased levels of lipids, including cholesterol, in the blood. If you already have hyperlipidaemia, because of type 2 diabetes, eating too much saturated fat will add to this problem. Mono- and polyunsaturated fats, on the other hand, do not have this effect on blood lipids and are the types of fats which can be used for essential chemical reactions in the body. It is particularly important, therefore, to make sure that the majority of the fats that you eat are mono- or polyunsaturated.

Sources of unsaturated fats – good!	Sources of saturated fats – bad!
Oily fish	Fatty meat
Nuts and seeds	Cheese
Sunflower, olive and rapeseed oils and spreads	Lard, suet
Avocados	Cream
Olives	Cakes, pastries

INCREASE YOUR ACTIVITY

Losing weight will also make it easier for you to get more exercise – you will be more mobile and have more energy. Exercising will help you to keep your weight off, and has numerous health benefits regardless of whether or not you are overweight. It will do wonders for your cardiovascular system, which is especially important given your increased risk of long-term problems in this area.

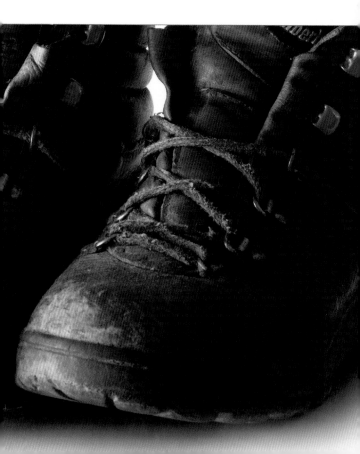

Some tips for leading a more active lifestyle include:

- Walk briskly for half-an-hour, five times a week.
- Choose stairs over lifts or escalators.
- Walk or cycle short journeys rather than using the car.
- Get out and about whenever possible – cut down on your time spent watching television or surfing the net!
- Encourage your family and friends to join you in a new active hobby – swimming or playing tennis, perhaps. Gyms often do special discounts for family membership.

STOP SMOKING

We all know that smoking is a very dangerous habit in terms of our health, but it is particularly dangerous if you have diabetes. You are already at increased risk of cardiovascular disease compared with people without diabetes, and if you smoke, this risk is increased further. Your GP or diabetes nurse will be able to advise you on how best to go about quitting, and offer you names of groups and helplines that you can contact for support.

	Two units (woman)	Three units (man)
Beer (ordinary strength)	1 pint	1.5 pints
Wine	2 small glasses	3 small glasses
Spirits	2 single measures	3 single measures
Sherry/fortified wine	2 small glasses	3 small glasses

DRINK ALCOHOL IN MODERATION

You may be surprised to hear that moderate alcohol consumption may actually improve your insulin sensitivity! However, too much alcohol, particularly on an empty stomach, can cause your blood sugar levels to drop dangerously low. Alcohol also stimulates your appetite and is high in calories, which won't complement a weight loss plan! So aim to drink in moderation only – two units of alcohol per day for a woman and three for a man.

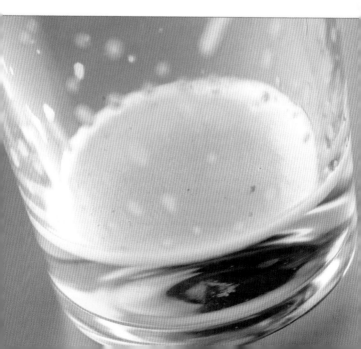

DRUG TREATMENT FOR TYPE 2 DIABETES

If your doctor decides that your lifestyle changes are not controlling your blood sugar level to an extent that he/she is happy with, they will 'step up' your treatment by prescribing you tablets. When deciding what drugs to give you to treat your type 2 diabetes, your doctor will be guided by national guidelines which have been set up by independent experts. Most doctors will refer to the National Institute for Health and Clinical Excellence (NICE) guidelines.

Even if you are given antidiabetic drugs, it is important that you continue to eat healthily, get plenty of exercise and stick to any weight-loss plans that you have agreed with your dietitian.

There are several different classes of antidiabetic drugs. Drugs are grouped into a single class if they act in the same way. Your doctor will take many factors into account in choosing which drug, or drugs, you will be treated with. The guidelines are quite specific in describing in what order these drugs should be tried. You may also be given more than one drug at the same time. One antidiabetic drug – Avandamet® – is actually a combination of two drugs in one product.

If you are prescribed drugs for your type 2 diabetes you will qualify for a prescription exemption certificate.

THE DIFFERENT TYPES OF ANTIDIABETIC DRUG

Drug class	Generic name	Brand names
Biguanides	Metformin	Glucophage®, Glucophage SR®, Glucamet®, Orabet®
Sulphonylureas	Chlorpropamide	–
	Glibenclamide	Daonil®, Semi-Daonil®, Euglucon®, Calabren®, Diabetamide®, Gliken®, Malix®
	Gliclazide	Diamicron®, Diamicron MR®, Diaglyk®, Vivazide®
	Glimepiride	Amaryl®
	Glipizide	Glibenese®, Minodiab®
	Gliquidone	Glurenorm®
	Tolbutamide	–
Prandial glucose regulators	Nateglinide	Starlix®
	Repaglinide	NovoNorm®
Thiazolidinediones	Pioglitazone	Actos®
	Rosiglitazone	Avandia® (and Avandamet® – combination drug containing rosiglitazone and metformin)
Alpha glucosidase inhibitors	Acarbose	Glucobay®

Drugs often have more than one name. A generic name, which refers to its active ingredient, and a brand name, which is the registered trade name given to it by the pharmaceutical company. Metformin is a generic name and Glucophage® is a brand name.

THE DRUG DEVELOPMENT PROCESS

Developing and launching a new drug onto the commercial market is an extremely costly and time-consuming venture. The process can take a pharmaceutical company between 10 and 15 years from the outset, at an estimated cost of £500 million. Much of this time is spent fulfilling strict guidelines set out by regulatory authorities in order to ensure the safety and quality of the end product. Once registered, a new drug is protected by a patent for 20 years, after which time other rival companies are free to manufacture and market identical drugs, called generics. Thus, the pharmaceutical company has a finite period of time before patent expiry to recoup the costs of drug development and return a profit to their shareholders.

During the development process, a drug undergoes five distinct phases of rigorous testing – the preclinical phase, which takes place in the laboratory – and phases 1, 2, 3 and 4, which involve testing in humans. Approval from the regulatory body and hence, a licence to sell the drug, is dependent on the satisfactory completion of all phases of testing. In the UK, the Medicines and Healthcare Products Regulatory Agency (MHRA) and the European Medicines Evaluation Agency (EMEA) regulate the drug development process.

- Only about 1 in every 100 drugs that enter the preclinical stage progress into human testing because they failed to work or had unacceptable side-effects.
- Animal testing is an important part of drug development. Before a drug reaches a human, it is vital that its basic safety has been established in an animal. Researchers do everything in their powers to minimise the number of animals they use and must adhere to strict guidelines issued by the Home Office.
- Phase 1 testing takes place in groups of 10–80 healthy volunteers.
- Phase 2 testing takes place in 100–300 patients diagnosed with the disease the drug is designed to treat.
- Phase 3 clinical trials involve between 1,000 and 3,000 patients with the relevant disease, and look at both the short- and long-term effects of the drug.
- Phase 4 testing and monitoring continues after the drug has reached the market.

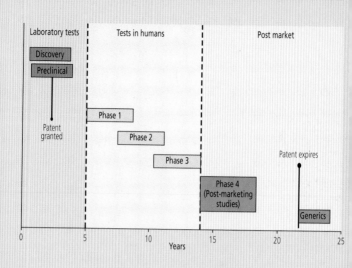

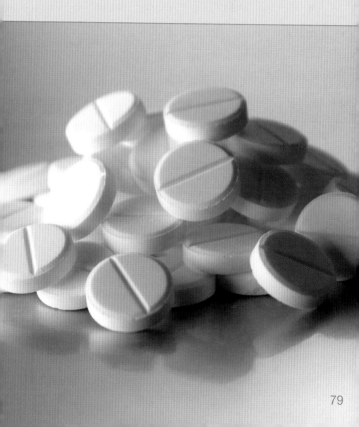

Biguanides

If you are overweight (with a BMI over 25 kg/m^2) and lifestyle changes have not brought your blood sugar levels under control, it is likely that your doctor will prescribe you metformin (Glucophage®, Glucophage SR®), which is the only biguanide drug available in the UK.

When metformin is the only antidiabetic drug you are using, you should not be at risk of your blood sugar level falling dangerously low (hypoglycaemia). This is because metformin does not increase the amount of insulin in the blood. Your doctor should perform regular blood tests to check that your kidneys are still working properly. He will also advise you if other drugs you are taking are likely to interfere with metformin.

Sulphonylureas

If you are not overweight, and your blood sugar level is not controlled despite a healthy, balanced diet, you may be prescribed a sulphonylurea drug by your doctor. These tablets are also offered to patients who would otherwise be taking metformin but cannot tolerate it. They may also be combined with metformin treatment in patients who do not show enough improvement with metformin on its own.

There is a risk that your blood sugar levels may fall to dangerously low levels during treatment with sulphonylureas, because they increase the amount of insulin in the blood.

Prandial glucose regulators

These drugs are used in the same groups of
patients as the sulphonylureas (those who are
not overweight, or those who are overweight
but cannot tolerate metformin). These drugs
carry a small risk of hypoglycaemia.

Thiazolidinediones (glitazones)

If you are overweight, and modifying your
lifestyle has not brought your blood sugar level
under control, but you are unable to take
metformin, you may be offered a glitazone.
Also, if either metformin or a sulphonylurea is
not adequately effective on its own and you
are not able to tolerate the combination of
both of them, thiazolidinediones may be used
to 'top up' either one or both, if your doctor
considers it appropriate. Rosiglitazone can
cause hypoglycaemia when used together with
sulphonylureas.

Alpha glucosidase inhibitors

One alternative drug (acarbose [Glucobay®]) is
available if you cannot tolerate any of the
other tablets which lower blood glucose, or if
the relevant combinations of those drugs have
not proven to be effective enough. Acarbose
can increase the risk of hypoglycaemia when
used together with sulphonylureas.

THE SIDE-EFFECTS MOST FREQUENTLY ASSOCIATED WITH ANTIDIABETIC DRUGS

Drug class	Risk of hypoglycaemia?	Common side-effects
Biguanides	Not usually	Mainly gastrointestinal (e.g. nausea, loss of appetite, vomiting, diarrhoea, abdominal pain); also metallic taste in mouth
Sulphonylureas	Yes	Mainly gastrointestinal, as for biguanides
Prandial glucose regulators	Yes	Itching and rashes; also gastrointestinal, as for biguanides
Thiazolidinediones (glitazones)	Rarely with pioglitazone, more commonly with rosiglitazone, both only when in combination with other oral antidiabetic agents.	Gastrointestinal, as for biguanides; also headache,
Alpha glucosidase inhibitors	May enhance hypoglycaemic effects of sulphonylureas	Problems with liver function, flatulence

If you experience symptoms which you think may be due to the medication you are taking, you should talk to your doctor, pharmacist or nurse. If the side-effect is unusual or severe, your GP may decide to report it to the Medicines and Healthcare Products Regulatory Agency (MHRA). The MHRA operates a 'Yellow Card Scheme' which is designed to flag up potentially dangerous drug effects and thereby protect patient safety. The procedure has changed recently to allow patients to report adverse drug reactions themselves. Visit www.yellowcard.gov.uk for more information.

HYPOGLYCAEMIA

If your blood sugar level falls below 4 mmol/L, you are considered to be hypoglycaemic.

If you suffer an episode of hypoglycaemia, or dangerously low blood sugar levels, it is important that you know exactly what to do. The action you need to take depends on the severity of the attack.

- **Mild hypoglycaemia** – treat with one of the following:
  - 10–30 g fast-acting carbohydrate (e.g. 3–6 glucose tablets)
  - 100 mL fizzy drink or squash (not the diet version!)
  - 100 mL milk
  - 50–100 mL Lucozade®
  - a drink containing two teaspoonfuls of sugar.

Follow this with some starchy carbohydrate, such as biscuits or bread, or a piece of fruit such as an apple or banana. Ensure that the next meal is also rich in carbohydrate (e.g. pasta or potatoes).

Chocolate is not very effective for treating hypoglycaemia. It does not release glucose very quickly – it has a relatively low GI rating, due to its fat content.

- **Moderate hypoglycaemia** – you may not be able to treat yourself if you have moderate hypoglycaemia. Make sure your friends and family know what to do in this situation. If you are conscious, the most effective treatment may be to use Hypostop Gel®. This is a thick gel, rich in glucose, which is given by mouth.

- **Severe hypoglycaemia** – if you are unconscious, you will need treatment with one of:
  - **glucagon** – a hormone which triggers glucose to be released from the liver, muscle and fat stores
  - **dextrose** – a form of glucose.

INSULIN THERAPY

If your blood sugar is still not controlled, your doctor may need to treat you with insulin injections. Your doctor may choose to give you insulin therapy even if you think that your blood sugar level is well controlled using other treatments. If you have complications such as neuropathy, or particularly if you have suffered a heart attack, you may benefit from insulin therapy.

Your doctor may well offer you insulin therapy in place of antidiabetic tablets. He may, on the other hand, treat you with a combination of insulin and antidiabetic tablets, a strategy which is thought to:

- make it easier for you to keep your weight down
- reduce your risk of hypoglycaemia

It is predicted that inhaled insulin will be available for the treatment of both type 1 and 2 diabetes during 2006.

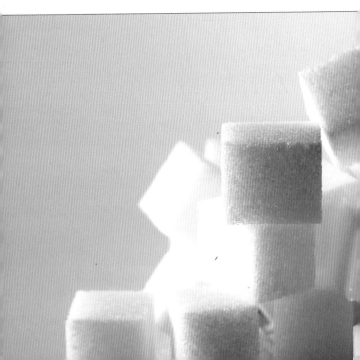

■ improve your control of blood sugar when
you first start receiving insulin therapy and
the best dose for you to take has not yet
been established.

Not all antidiabetic drugs can be taken
together with insulin therapy, so your doctor
will decide whether or not to combine
different treatments.

If it were taken in a tablet form, insulin
would be broken down by the acid in the
stomach. Therefore, it is injected
subcutaneously (literally, 'under the skin'),
either using a 'pen' device or a syringe. Pens
may be prefilled, or may be reusable, with
insulin supplied in cartridges.

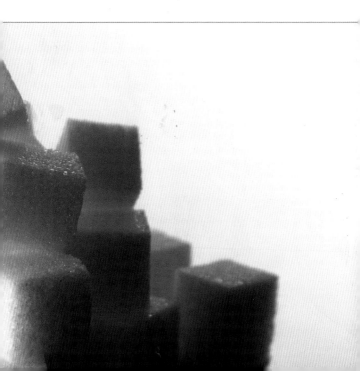

ANTIOBESITY DRUGS FOR TYPE 2 DIABETES

If you have lost some weight by modifying your diet and exercise patterns, and yet you remain overweight, your doctor may consider it appropriate to offer you a drug to aid your attempts to lose weight. The drugs available in the UK for this purpose are:

- orlistat (Xenical®)
- sibutramine hydrochloride (Reductil®).

TREATMENT OF HIGH BLOOD PRESSURE

Approximately half of people with type 2 diabetes also have high blood pressure. Your doctor will therefore monitor your blood pressure at regular intervals and treat hypertension if it occurs, to keep your blood pressure below 140/80 mmHg. The lifestyle changes that you are making will help to reduce your blood pressure, but a number of drugs are also available for this purpose:

- thiazide diuretics (e.g. indapamide [Natrilix®, Natrilix SR®] and xipamide [Diurexan®])
- beta-blockers (e.g. propranolol [Inderal®] and acebutolol [Sectral®])
- angiotensin-converting enzyme (ACE) inhibitors (e.g. captopril [Capoten®] and enalapril [Innovace®])
- calcium-channel blockers (e.g. isradipine [Prescal®] and lacidipine [Motens®])
- angiotensin II receptor blockers (e.g. irbesartan [Aprovel®] and losartan [Cozaar®]).

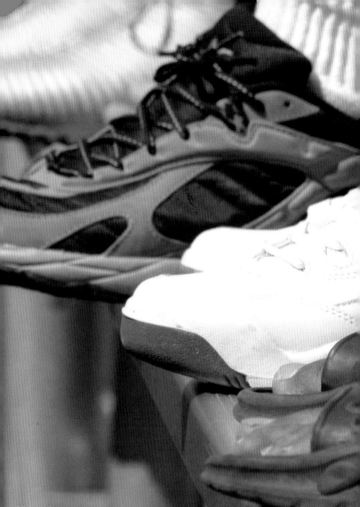

REGULAR EXERCISE IS AN IMPORTANT PART OF ANY WEIGHT-LOSS PROGRAMME.

For more information on the drugs used to manage blood pressure refer to A Simple Guide to Blood Pressure.

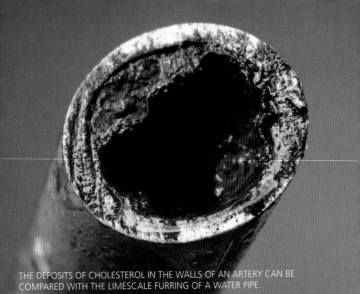

THE DEPOSITS OF CHOLESTEROL IN THE WALLS OF AN ARTERY CAN BE COMPARED WITH THE LIMESCALE FURRING OF A WATER PIPE.

THE COMPLICATIONS ASSOCIATED WITH TYPE 2 DIABETES

The risk of complications increases the longer you have type 2 diabetes. Remember, though, that you may have had type 2 diabetes for some time without knowing it, so be on the look out for signs of complications as soon as you are diagnosed.

CORONARY HEART DISEASE AND STROKE

For more information on cardiovascular disease and its risk factors, refer to *A Simple Guide to Cholesterol*.

If you have type 2 diabetes, then the lipid content of your blood is high. This can lead to the build up of fatty deposits inside your blood vessels. If this happens, your blood vessels will begin to get narrower and they may eventually become blocked, leading to a heart attack or a stroke. People with type 2 diabetes are at greater risk of developing coronary heart disease than people with normal blood sugar levels.

What to look out for

As well as the more common features of cardiovascular disease (e.g. shortness of breath, irregular heartbeat, chest pain), cardiovascular disease caused by diabetes has an odd feature that is worth being aware of. Because type 2 diabetes causes nerve damage (called diabetic neuropathy), you might be less likely to feel pain and discomfort. Therefore you might not experience the main warning sign – chest pain. People with diabetes may even suffer a heart attack without feeling any pain – a 'silent heart attack'. In place of chest pain, you might experience:

- nausea
- sweating
- light-headedness
- vomiting
- breathlessness.

What can be done about it?

The good news is that the lifestyle modifications that you have been advised to make for the management of your type 2 diabetes will also reduce your risk of cardiovascular disease.

You may also be given drugs to reduce the lipid content of your blood (e.g. statins).

A stroke occurs when the brain is starved of oxygen because its blood supply is interrupted.

DIABETIC RETINOPATHY AND CATARACTS

Diabetic retinopathy is a serious eye condition that can cause loss of vision. If blood sugar levels remain high over a long period of time, they can damage the tiny blood vessels that supply the retina. The vessels get bigger, and start to leak fluid. They may even break and cause bleeding.

There are three types of diabetic retinopathy.

■ **Background/simple retinopathy** – this is the most common form of retinopathy. It only involves mild damage to the blood vessels and is not threatening to sight but should be closely monitored.

■ **Maculopathy** – the mild damage which occurs in background retinopathy affects the area of the retina which is used most, and is needed for clear, detailed vision (the

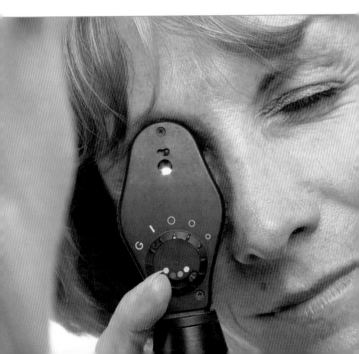

macula). The centre of your vision gradually deteriorates, but the surrounding regions (peripheral vision) shouldn't be affected.

■ **Proliferative retinopathy** – some of the blood vessels to the retina are damaged to such an extent that they become blocked completely. New ones start to develop to replace them. There will probably be bleeding, and scar tissue may develop which can pull the retina out of position. This condition causes vision to deteriorate, and if it is left untreated, may result in blindness.

A cataract is a clouding over of the lens of the eye, which interferes with vision. Cataracts tend to occur at younger ages in people who have diabetes.

What to look out for

It is vital to have regular eye checks, which might be carried out by your GP, your consultant diabetologist or an optometrist/optician. These eye examinations should be carried out every year.

What can be done about it?

In its early stages, damage to the eyes caused by diabetes may actually be reversed if blood pressure and blood sugar are rigorously controlled. However, once retinopathy reaches the more severe stages of maculopathy, laser treatment can be used to prevent further damage (though it does not repair the damage that is already done). The procedure is performed under a local anaesthetic.

DIABETIC NEUROPATHY

Diabetic neuropathy is a serious disease in which nerves become permanently damaged. There are several ways that nerve damage occurs as a result of diabetes, but one involves damage to blood vessels, similar to that which occurs in diabetic retinopathy. If the vessels which carry blood to nerves are damaged by excessive amounts of glucose, the nerves do not receive enough oxygen, and can become damaged or even die off. The form of neuropathy most relevant to diabetes is called peripheral neuropathy. It affects the extremities, such as the feet, hands, legs and arms.

What to look out for

To start with you would usually experience numbness, tingling or pain in your feet. The nerves which supply your feet are the longest in your body, and so these are usually the first to be affected by neuropathy.

Make sure you tell your doctor if you experience these symptoms. If he suspects that you might have diabetic neuropathy, he will probably examine your feet thoroughly, and carry out a range of tests to determine your nerve and muscle function. If your feet become affected by peripheral neuropathy, your GP will refer you to a chiropodist.

What can be done about it?

Develop a regular foot care routine and put it into action straight away.

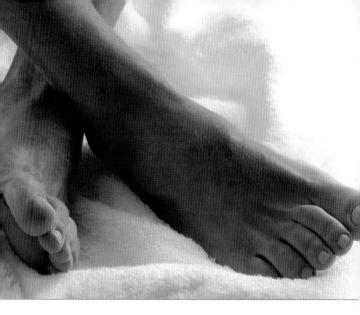

- Clean your feet daily in warm water, drying them thoroughly afterwards.
- Inspect them carefully for blisters, ulcers, cuts, redness, calluses or swelling.
- Moisturise your feet (except between your toes).
- After washing your feet, file any corns or calluses with a pumice stone.
- Cut your toenails at least once a week.
- Never wear shoes that fit poorly or are damaged inside.
- Always wear shoes or slippers, even indoors, to protect your feet from injury.

You should also have an annual foot examination carried out by a doctor, nurse or chiropodist. If you do develop serious problems with your feet, you may be admitted to hospital for the treatment of ulcers, or be given antibiotics if you have an infection.

DIABETIC NEPHROPATHY

When they are working properly, the kidneys filter harmful chemicals out of the blood, but ensure that the proteins which are needed in the body are not lost into the urine. Diabetic nephropathy is a condition in which the kidneys become increasingly 'leaky' to proteins which should be retained in the blood. The high blood pressure associated with diabetes is largely responsible for this, but high blood glucose levels can also affect the membranes in the kidneys which are responsible for filtering the blood. Not only are proteins lost to the urine when they shouldn't be, but the kidneys can also lose their ability to filter out harmful chemicals from the blood. The build-up of these chemicals in the blood represents the most dangerous problem in nephropathy, and can be fatal if left untreated.

There are three stages of diabetic nephropathy.

- **Microalbuminuria** – small amounts of protein leaked into urine.
- **Proteinuria** – larger amounts of protein leaked into urine. Kidneys begin to lose their ability to filter potentially harmful chemicals out of the blood.
- **End-stage kidney/renal disease** – kidneys function very poorly. Potentially harmful chemicals in the blood can build up to fatal levels.

What to look out for

The main symptom that you may notice is swelling of your feet and legs, progressing to other areas of the body. Other symptoms may include fatigue, nausea, itchy skin and heartburn. As part of your normal management programme, you will be receiving regular checks of your blood pressure as well as tests for protein in your urine, so any changes should be detected early.

The boundaries for diagnosis of nephropathy by the amount of protein in a urine sample are:

Diagnosis	Amount of protein
Normal	Less than 30 milligrams
Microalbuminuria	30–300 milligrams
Proteinuria	Over 300 milligrams

What can be done about it?

High blood pressure is the main culprit responsible for diabetic nephropathy. Therefore, when there is a significant amount of protein in your urine, the first treatment you are likely to receive is medication that will lower your blood pressure. You may also be advised to pay particular attention to reducing the protein content in your diet (contained in foods such as meat, dairy products, pulses and nuts, for example). If you progress as far as end-stage renal disease you will require kidney dialysis (which means that your blood is artificially filtered, instead of relying on the kidney to do this) and may be given a kidney transplant.

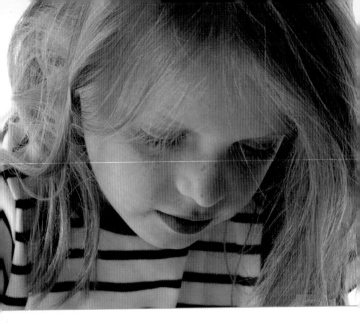

SPECIAL CASES

Children

Type 2 diabetes in children is still quite rare. When it does occur, the same dietary and lifestyle modifications that are advised for adults apply. It is a good idea to inform the child's school about their diabetes, so that they can make the appropriate allowances (e.g. allowing for frequent visits to the toilet).

Although metformin is licensed for use in children over the age of 10 years, most other antidiabetic treatments are not advisable for children. The risk of developing complications of type 2 diabetes increases the longer the duration of the disease, so people who develop type 2 diabetes at a young age are at a particularly high risk of these complications later in life. Thus, establishing good control of blood sugar at an early stage is of the utmost importance in children.

Pregnancy

If you have type 2 diabetes, it is perfectly possible for you to have a safe and healthy pregnancy. Because of your condition, however, you will need to plan your pregnancy carefully. The first few weeks of your pregnancy are particularly important in terms of your baby's health, and so it is important that your blood sugar is well controlled prior to conception. If you are taking antidiabetic tablets, you will need to switch to insulin therapy during your pregnancy.

Most diabetes-related problems during pregnancy tend to arise from hyperglycaemia rather than hypoglycaemia. Excessive blood sugar levels during pregnancy can lead the baby to grow abnormally large (which may necessitate a Caesarean section), as well as to high blood pressure in the mother and hypoglycaemia in the baby at birth. As you know, a risk for developing type 2 diabetes can be inherited, and there may be an increased chance of your baby developing type 2 diabetes (or being overweight) in later life.

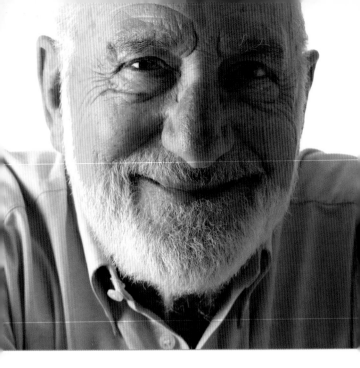

Elderly

If you are elderly, you may find it more difficult to make lifestyle changes than younger patients. If you need insulin therapy, you may find that age-related problems such as arthritis and visual impairment make insulin injections more difficult.

Elderly people are particularly vulnerable to hypoglycaemia, and it can also be more difficult to recognise. In order to reduce your risk of hypoglycaemic attacks, your doctor may relax your treatment a little in order to keep your blood sugar controlled at a slightly higher level than would be aimed for in younger patients. Metformin is a useful drug in elderly patients as it does not generally cause hypoglycaemia.

DIETARY SUPPLEMENTATION FOR TYPE 2 DIABETES

Aside from the recognised treatment options that we have already looked at, there are a number of dietary supplements that you may wish to consider. The use of these supplements tends to be supported more by belief than by rigorous scientific testing. Whatever you are using to manage your type 2 diabetes, you must be sure to inform your doctor. Some supplements may interfere with the way your other treatments work, and so your doctor needs to know about them.

Dietary supplements are not tested in the same way as drugs, and so their safety is not known.

Herbs and spices thought to contribute to good diabetes control include:

- cinnamon – to improve glucose uptake into cells and reduce blood lipids
- fenugreek – to improve glucose uptake into cells
- garlic – to lower blood lipids
- *Salacia oblonga* – to reduce blood sugar
- *Ginko biloba* extracts – for early-stage diabetic neuropathy.

TYPE 2 DIABETES AND DRIVING

If your blood sugar levels are not well controlled and you are at risk of hypoglycaemia, it can be very dangerous to drive, as this can make you lose concentration or even consciousness. Because hypoglycaemia is a risk associated with insulin treatment and some antidiabetic tablets, the way in which your diabetes is being treated determines whether you should inform the Driver and Vehicle Licensing Agency (DVLA).

- If you are using only **lifestyle changes** to manage your condition, no restrictions will be imposed on your driving as long as your eyesight remains adequate. You need not inform the DVLA at this stage.
- If you are taking **antidiabetic tablets**, you must inform the DVLA of your condition,

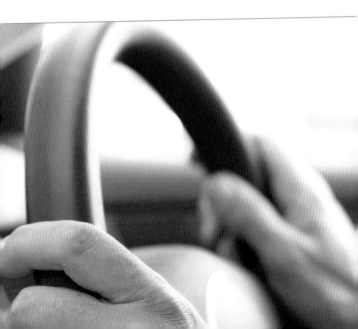

but again, no restrictions are likely to be imposed as long as your eyesight is good enough (see *www.dvla.gov.uk*).

■ If you are being treated with insulin, you must inform the DVLA, and your driving license will be altered so that it needs to be renewed every 3 years. At this stage, you may also be prevented from driving larger vehicles (over 3.5 tonnes or with more than eight seats).

■ No matter how your condition is being managed (even if by lifestyle modification alone), you must inform your driving insurance company.

There are a number of precautions you can take to avoid hypoglycaemic attacks whilst driving.

■ Check your blood sugar level before you leave.

■ Try to break for a snack every couple of hours if you are travelling a long distance.

■ Keep a sugary food or drink in the car (e.g. glucose tablets) for if you begin to feel hypoglycaemic.

■ Work your journey around meal times so that you don't have to change them.

It is also a good idea to carry some identification in the car with you, explaining that you have type 2 diabetes, in case you do suffer a hypoglycaemic attack and need help from a stranger. If you tend to have difficulty recognising the early signs of a hypoglycaemic attack, it is probably best to avoid driving altogether.

THE LONG AND SHORT OF IT

What should I expect?

Type 2 diabetes is a long-term condition, and unfortunately, once it is properly established, it cannot be cured. However, if managed well, type 2 diabetes should not restrict your daily life - the management process actually involves adopting a more healthy, active lifestyle. There is a range of effective treatment options and a team of healthcare professionals available to help you manage your condition properly.

The term 'diabetes' often conjures up an image of a life dependent on insulin injections. If you have type 2 diabetes, insulin injections are just one of the treatment options and, even if you are prescribed them, you may not need them for the rest of your life.

Why does it need to be treated?

The symptoms of type 2 diabetes emerge gradually, and may not even be very troublesome. You may question whether to bother making an effort to manage your condition effectively. The important thing to remember is that, if poorly managed, type 2 diabetes can lead to a range of unpleasant and potentially serious complications. Achieving good control of your diabetes in the short term significantly reduces your risk of being troubled by these complications in the future.

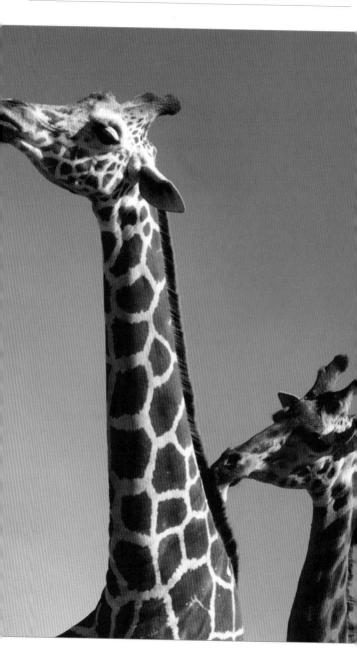

BECOMING AN EXPERT PATIENT

Diabetes is a long-term disease that usually affects you for the rest of your life. People with diabetes may benefit from joining the Expert Patient Programme, run by the NHS. The scheme is aimed at encouraging people with long-term health conditions to take more control over their health by understanding and managing their conditions. By enrolling on the Expert Patient Programme you will ultimately be able to use your skills and knowledge to lead a fuller life. Courses take 6 weeks to complete and are run throughout the country. Visit *www.expertpatients.nhs.uk* for more information.

FIVE STEPS TO GETTING THE MOST OUT OF YOUR HEALTH SERVICE

1 Maintain a good relationship with your GP and the other members of your team.

2 Keep your team informed of any changes you notice in your symptoms.

3 Keep your team informed of all the treatments you are taking, including dietary supplements.

4 Agree with your team on your personal management targets.

5 Know what to expect and when you need to ask for help.

GETTING THE MOST OUT OF YOUR HEALTH SERVICE

Type 2 diabetes is a long-term (or chronic) condition, and each case needs to be treated individually. There are steps you can take to ensure that your own case of diabetes is managed as well as it can be.

Having a doctor's appointment or attending a clinic can be a daunting prospect. You may find that your consultation or clinic is led very much by the doctor or nurse and when they ask you if you have any questions, your mind goes blank. It is often helpful to write down a list of questions before you attend your appointment or the clinic.

Make sure you are aware of your personal targets at each stage of your treatment, as agreed by your care team:

■ ideal weight
■ target blood/urine glucose level
■ target HbA_{1C}
■ target blood pressure
■ target cholesterol
■ alcohol limits
■ amount of exercise.

Although you cannot monitor all of these targets yourself at home, be aware of what values you are aiming for.

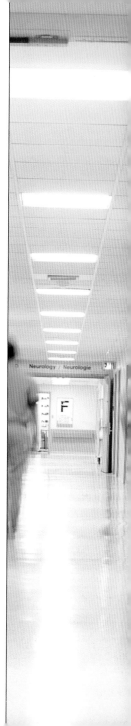

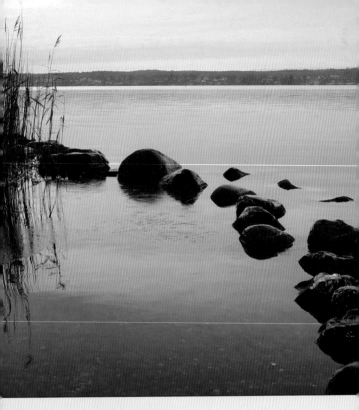

QUESTIONS TO ASK YOUR DOCTOR

- How serious is type 2 diabetes?
- Will I be treated with tablets or insulin straight away?
- How often should I come in for check-ups/clinics?
- What signs should I look out for with respect to the complications of type 2 diabetes?
- What will happen if I don't take my medication?
- How often and at what times should I take my antidiabetic tablets?
- How and when should I inject my insulin?
- What should my family know? Should they attend clinics or appointments with me?
- Can I still drive?
- I am planning to get pregnant. What preparations should I make?

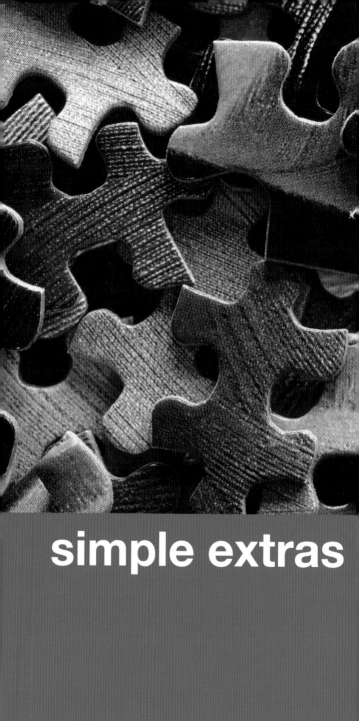

simple extras

FURTHER READING

- *www.committogetfit.com*
- *www.healthyliving.gov.uk*
- *www.eatwell.gov.uk*
- *www.weightlossresources.co.uk*
- *Balance* – a bi-monthly magazine, available from newsagents or free to members of Diabetes UK.

USEFUL CONTACTS

- **Action on Smoking and Health**
  Tel: 020 7739 5902
  Website: *www.ash.org.uk*

- **Association for the Study of Obesity**
  Website: *www.aso.org.uk*

- **British Heart Foundation**
  14 Fitzhardinge Street
  London
  W1H 6DH
  Tel: 020 7935 0185
  Email: *internet@bhf.org.uk*
  Website: *www.bhf.org.uk*

- **Diabetes Research and Wellness Foundation**
  101-102 Northney Marina
  Hayling Island
  Hampshire
  PO11 0NH
  Tel: 023 92 637 808
  Fax: 023 92 636 137
  Website: *www.diabeteswellnessnet.org.uk*

■ **Diabetes UK**
Central office
10 Parkway
London
NW1 7AA
Tel: 020 7424 1000
Email: *info@diabetes.org.uk*
Website: *www.diabetes.org.uk*

■ **Driver and Vehicle Licensing Agency (DVLA)**
The Medical Adviser
Drivers Medical Unit
DVLA
Longview Road
Swansea
SA99 1TU
Tel: 01792 772151
Website: *www.dvla.gov.uk/welcome.htm*

■ **International Diabetic Athletes Association**
Website: *www.diabetes-exercise.org*

■ **International Diabetes Federation (IDF)**
Avenue Emile De Mot 19
B-1000 Brussels
Belgium
Tel: 00 32 2 5385511
Website: *www.idf.org*

■ **National Institute for Health and Clinical Excellence (NICE)**
11 The Strand
London
WC2N 5HR
Tel. 020 7766 9191
Website: *www.nice.org.uk/nice-web*

■ **National Kidney Research Fund**
Registered Office
Kings Chambers
Priestgate
Peterborough
PE1 1FG
Tel: 0845 070 7601
Website: *www.nkrf.org.uk/index.htm*

■ **Neuropathy Trust**
Website: *www.neuropathy-trust.org/index.htm*

■ **NHS Direct**
NHS Direct Line: 0845 4647
Website: *www.nhsdirect.nhs.uk*

■ **The Patients Association**
PO BOX 935
Harrow
Middlesex
HA1 3YJ
Tel: 020 8423 9111
Helpline: 08456 08 4455
Website: *www.patients-association.com*

■ **Royal National Institute of the Blind**
105 Judd Street
London
WC1H 9NE
Tel: 020 7388 1266
Website: *www.rnib.org.uk*

■ **Weight Watchers UK**
Website: *www.weightwatchers.co.uk*

YOUR RIGHTS

As a patient, you have a number of important rights. These include the right to the best possible standard of care, the right to information, the right to dignity and respect, the right to confidentiality and underpinning all of these, the right to good health.

Occasionally, you may feel as though your rights have been compromised, or you may be unsure of where you stand when it comes to qualifying for certain treatments or services. In these instances, there are a number of organisations you can turn to for help and advice. Remember that lodging a complaint against your health service should not compromise the quality of care you receive, either now or in the future.

■ **Patients Association**
The Patients Association (*www.patients-association.com*) is a UK charity which represents patient rights, influences health policy and campaigns for better patient care.
Contact details:
PO Box 935
Harrow
Middlesex
HA1 3YJ
Helpline: 08456 084455
Email: *mailbox@patients-association.com*

■ **Citizens Advice Bureau**
The Citizens Advice Bureau (*www.nacab.org.uk*) provides free, independent and confidential advice to NHS patients at a number of outreach centres located throughout the country (*www.adviceguide.org.uk*).
Contact details:
Find your local Citizens Advice Bureau using the search tool at *www.citizensadvice.org.uk*

- **Patient Advice and Liaison Services (PALS)**
  Set up by the Department of Health (*www.dh.gov.uk*), PALS
  provide information, support and confidential advice to patients,
  families and their carers.
  Contact details:
  Phone your local hospital, clinic, GP surgery or health centre and
  ask for details of the PALS, or call NHS Direct on 0845 46 47.

- **The Independent Complaints Advocacy Service (ICAS)**
  ICAS is an independent service that can help you bring about
  formal complaints against your NHS practitioner. ICAS provides
  support, help, advice and advocacy from experienced advisors
  and caseworkers.
  Contact details:
  ICAS Central Team
  Myddelton House
  115–123 Pentonville Road
  London N1 9LZ
  Email: *icascentralteam@citizensadvice.org.uk*
  Or contact your local ICAS office direct.

Accessing your medical records

You have a legal right to see all your health records under the Data
Protection Act of 1998. You can usually make an informal request to
your doctor and you should be given access within 40 days. Note
that you may have to pay a small fee for the privilege.

You can be denied access to your records if your doctor believes
that the information contained within them could cause serious
harm to you or another person. If you are applying for access on
behalf of someone else, then you will not be granted access to
information which the patient gave to his or her doctor on the
understanding that it would remain confidential.

PERSONAL RECORD:

My Simple Guide

This Simple Guide to Type 2 Diabetes belongs to:

Name:

Address:

Tel No:

Email:

In case of emergency please contact:

Name:

Address:

Tel No:

Email:

My Healthcare Team

GP surgery address and telephone number

Name:

Address:

Tel No:

I am registered with Dr

My practice nurse

My endocrinologist

My pharmacist

Other members of my healthcare team

QUESTIONS

_____

_____

_____

_____

_____

_____

_____

_____

_____

_____

_____

_____

_____

_____

_____

ANSWERS

NOTES

_____

_____

_____

_____

_____

_____

_____

_____

_____

_____

_____

_____

_____

_____

_____

_____